CARE

Human Care and Health Series

General Editor

Madeleine M. Leininger, R.N., M.S.N., L.H.D., Ph.D., F.A.A.N.
Professor of Nursing and Adjunct Professor of Anthropology
Colleges of Nursing and Liberal Arts
Wayne State University

National Advisory Review Board

CARE

THE ESSENCE OF NURSING AND HEALTH

Edited by

Madeleine M. Leininger, R.N., Ph.D., L.H.D., F.A.A.N.

WAYNE STATE UNIVERSITY PRESS   DETROIT   1988

Library of Congress Cataloging-in-Publication Data

Care, the essence of nursing and health / edited by Madeleine M.
   Leininger.
      p. cm. — (Human care and health series)
      Reprint. Originally published: Thorofare, NJ: Slack, c 1984.
      Includes bibliographies and index.
      ISBN 0-8143-1994-7. ISBN 0-8143-1995-5 (pbk.)
      1. Nursing—Psychological aspects. 2. Nursing—Philosophy.
   3. Caring. I. Leininger, Madeleine M. II. Series.
      [DNLM: 1. Nursing Care. 2. Philosophy, Nursing. WY 86 L531c
   1984a]
   RT86.C36 1988
   610.73'01—dc19
                                                               87-30043
                                                                    CIP

CONTENTS

Part Two: Research and Application to Nursing (Cont'd)

PREFACE

Today's thinking and findings influence tomorrow's decisions, plans, and actions. This statement has meaning if nurses will take a committed and active stance to make care the dominant and unifying focus of nursing. Care is a worthy area in which to discover the scientific and humanistic nature of nursing. An awareness of and sensitivity to care, backed by systematic investigations of care phenomena, offer one of the greatest hopes for improving health care services to advance the discipline of nursing.

While there is a committed core of nurse scholars and researchers studying care, the numbers are still very small when one considers that there are nearly four thousand nurse-researchers and four million professional nurses in the world. What would happen if all nurse-researchers were truly committed to studying and practicing care? What would happen if nurse theoreticians focused primarily on therapeutic care outcomes rather than energy, temporality, environment, and other secondary concepts? What would happen if care had a high economic value? What would happen if therapeutic care was publicly recognized and rewarded in the mass media? If these questions were addressed with resultant positive outcomes, one could predict that both scientific and humanistic aspects of care might well revolutionize future health care systems and educational programs.

The reality is that care remains a largely unknown and covert component of professional health services. It is like a rough diamond yet to be polished to expose its brilliant facets. Care, however, is the factor that appears to make the difference in human health services for well and sick people. There are multiple aspects of care that need to be fully explicated for the many subtle and largely covert factors related to therapeutic or nontherapeutic outcomes. Identifying and understanding the relationship of care to healing, curing, and health promotion is of much interest to care researchers and clinicians.

A *science of care* is needed to understand and value the nature of care in all its different meanings and expressions. The specific and universal aspects of care must continue to be studied. When I began the first cross-cultural study of care in the early 1960s, I was pleased to discover that cultures were able to identify care components as an important value in living. Since then, several transcultural nurses have focused on comparative care as the central and unique domain of nursing. As a consequence, a body of transcultural care knowledge has greatly influenced the study of care in the United States. There are, however, many cultures to be studied regarding care.

It is encouraging that consumers tend to view nurses as care providers, but the role attributes remain vague and are often misunderstood with curative medical regimens. It is of concern that not all professional nurses value care and use care theory and knowledge to guide nursing decisions and actions. Some nurses have drifted away from the practice of care. It is time to help nurses and future nursing students know, understand, and value care as the essence and unique aspect of nursing. It is time to discover the many unknown components of care. It is also time to institutionalize care as a *normative value* of nursing and other human health services. This reinforces these goals to make care the heart and essence of nursing.

This is the second major book on care. The first book, *Caring: An Essential Human Need,* was published in 1981 and has already influenced many nurses to rethink the value and importance of care. Many of the care experts in the field have shared their philosophic, theoretic, and research viewpoints about care. Their contributions reflect the serious attention they have given to care for more than a decade.

The first part of the book contains the original work of the contributors regarding the theoretic, philosophic, and conceptual dimensions of care. The second part of the book focuses on specific care research studies and their application to nursing and health practices. These chapters are intellectually stimulating to students of care. The authors are the leaders who stimulate nurses and others to study care systematically and make it the essence and unique feature of nursing. The authors' different perspectives about care phenomena based upon their research, theoretic, and philosophic study makes the book a valuable teaching and research document. Some of the thinking of the contributors came from the National Research Caring Conferences which have been held since 1976. The National Transcultural Nursing Care Conferences have also focused on comparative caring phenomena, which have influenced much of the writer's thinking and research.

The reader will find many ideas about care discussed by the authors. These ideas should stimulate the serious student of care to take hold of ideas that need further study, and it should challenge the lethargic student of care to get involved in care processes and practices. The ideas, theories, and research findings in this book should also lead to some significant and major curriculum, teaching, and research changes in nursing. For if nurses want to be known as care providers and advocates, then they must become knowledgeable about care. Nurses must be enculturated or socialized into a care ethnos and care practices. Care should become the organizing and central focus of the nursing profession. Nursing service, faculty, and administrators need to study and use care as a viable reality. When humanistic and scientific care becomes fully realized and practiced in nursing, then nursing will become a full-fledged and valued discipline and profession. It is hoped that by the year 2000, nurses will have a body of knowledge to support nursing care practices.

In general, the reader should find that this book offers valuable content about care. It is a comprehensive and scholarly treatise on the phenomenon of care based upon a number of research studies. These ideas and conceptualizations of care should help move nurses to recognize their role in the use of care constructs and to give new hope for nursing's distinct attributes. Colleagues from other disciplines interested in care will find areas of congruence in thinking as well as areas that need further interdisciplinary dialogue and research. It is indeed one of the most comprehensive and stimulating treatises on care, especially from a nursing and general human service viewpoint.

ACKNOWLEDGMENTS

I wish to acknowledge with deep appreciation the core of creative scholars, researchers, teachers, and leaders who have pioneered with me for more than a decade to make care a visible, dominant, and central focus of nursing knowledge and practice. I am especially grateful to Dr. Agnes Aamodt, Dr. Joyceen Boyle, Dr. Delores Gaut, Kathryn Gardner, Winnifred Gustafson, Dr. Peggy Field, Malcolm MacDonald, Em Bevis, Joyce Murray, Dr. Marilyn Ray, Dr. Michael Higgins, Doris Riemen, Joan Uhl, Dr. Janet Wang, and Dr. Jean Watson, who have maintained an active interest in care phenomena and have shared their ideas with other colleagues at the National Research Caring and Transcultural Nursing Conferences in the past decade.

I am also grateful to my own caring family who continue to be most supportive of my academic and professional work.

CONTRIBUTORS

Agnes M. Aamodt, RN, MSN, PhD, FAAN
Professor of Nursing
Division Coordinator, Maternal-Child Nursing
College of Nursing
University of Arizona
Tucson, AZ

Joyceen S. Boyle, RN, MPH, PhD
Associate Professor of Nursing
College of Nursing
University of Utah
Salt Lake City, UT

Anna Baziak Dugan, RN, MSN, MA, PhD
Associate Professor of Nursing
College of Nursing
Wayne State University
Detroit, MI

Fran Farrell, RN, MSW
Tucson, AZ

Peggy-Anne Field, RN, SCM, PhD
Professor of Nursing
Faculty of Nursing
University of Alberta
Edmonton, Alberta, Canada

Delores A. Gaut, RN, MS, PhD
Assistant Professor of Parent and Child Nursing
School of Nursing
University of Washington
Seattle, WA

Suellen Grassl-Herwehe, RN, MSN
Associate Faculty
Pima Community College
Tucson, AZ

Winnifred Gustafson, RN, MS
Assistant Professor of Nursing
School of Nursing
University of Wisconsin-Superior
Superior, WI

John Hutter Jr, MD
Associate Professor of Pediatrics
Section of Pediatric Hematology-Oncolgy
University of Arizona Health Science Center
Tucson, AZ

Madeleine M. Leininger, RN, MSN, PhD, LhD, FAAN
Professor of Nursing and Anthropology
Director, Center for Health Research
College of Nursing
Wayne State University
Detroit, MI

Malcolm MacDonald, RN, MN, EdD
Chairman, Nursing and Allied Health Division
Director, Nursing Programs
Cuesta College
San Luis Obispo, CA

Mary Sue Mennen Moore, RN, MS
Instructor
The University of Texas Health Science Center
San Antonio School of Nursing
San Antonio, TX

Marilyn A. Ray, RN, MSN, PhD
Nurse Researcher
College of Nurses of Ontario
Toronto, Ontario, Canada

Janet F. Wang, RN, PhD
Assistant Professor
School of Nursing
West Virginia University
Morgantown, WV

Cynthia J. Weiss, RN, MS, PhD
Assistant Professor of Nursing
Regional Campuses Associate Degree in Nursing Program
Kent State University
Ashtabula Campus
Ashtabula, OH

PART ONE: Philosophic, Theoretic and General Conceptualizations of Care

1

Care: The Essence
of Nursing and Health

For several decades, the author has taken a philosophic, theoretic, and research posture that *care is the essence and the central, unifying, and dominant domain to characterize nursing.*[1-4] Care has also been postulated to be an *essential human need for the full development, health maintenance, and survival of human beings in all world cultures.*[4] These statements are provocative and challenge nurses and the nursing profession. They are stimulating new lines of systematic investigation about care.

It is amazing that complacent attitudes about the importance of care as the essence of nursing and as an essential to health care can still be found. While there are signs of general interest on the parts of professionals and the public, care has not yet received the same degree of attention as cure. Why has there been a cultural lag in studying and focusing on care? Why does the public media give far more attention to dramatic medical (physician) cures than to nursing care? What cultural, social, political, and professional factors tend to influence the dominant trend toward cure and so limited emphasis on care? Most assuredly, physician curing modes receive far more attention than nursing care modes. As a consequence, there are more research monies for cure than for care research, and thus, more financial support for curing than caring activities.

Many speculative questions concerning this worldwide problem exist. For example, does cure receive more attention than care because cure has been traditionally associated with males who get public recognition for their efforts? The public tends to reinforce dramatic cures that use new technologies, diagnostic tools, and physical modes of treatment. Such new methods of cure generally receive high "payoffs" and receive quick recognition in the national or international public media. In contrast, females throughout history have provided many kinds of caring to individuals, families, and groups of people. Generally, nurses know the importance and positive benefits of care. Many professional female nurses have traditionally provided exquisite caring behaviors such as compassion, support, and comfort. They are generally aware that

3

care is important to client recovery. Why are these important nursing care processes and activities not recognized and valued as equally by the public as the emphasized physician cure practices? Are care and cure primarily sex-linked issues?

Such a line of inquiry about care and cure is important, but other areas also need systematic investigation. Care research deserves public emphasis in order to explicate and use the essential attributes of care for human growth, development, healing processes, and survival. Care research is indeed a neglected area of study and one that could potentially revolutionize the quality of health services in the world.

In this chapter, I discuss the general importance of care and health, and the need for nurses, the nursing profession, and the public to give more attention to these phenomena. It is essential to human health and is the unique and major feature that distinguishes nursing from other disciplines. Some of the critical issues in care and factors why it has not been given systematic, rigorous, and widespread investigation in nursing are identified. Emphasis is also given to making care a dominant transcultural or worldwide focus in nursing theory in order to help nurses understand and deal with it in all research, teaching, and practice endeavors.

CLARIFICATION OF THE TERMS: CARE, CARING, AND ESSENCE

Several terms need to be clarified at the outset.

Care in a generic sense refers to those assistive, supportive, or facilitative acts toward or for another individual or group with evident or anticipated needs to ameliorate or improve a human condition or lifeway.[4]

Caring refers to the direct (or indirect) nurturant and skillful activities, processes, and decisions related to assisting people in such a manner that reflects behavioral attributes which are empathetic, supportive, compassionate, protective, succorant, educational, and others dependent upon the needs, problems, values, and goals of the individual or group being assisted.[4]

Essence refers to a necessary constituent or an essential attribute which makes a thing or act what it is.[5]

Health refers to a state of well being that is mainly known and expressed in cultural meanings and ways.

Nursing refers to a learned humanistic art and science that focuses upon personalized (individual and group) care behaviors, functions, and processes directed toward promoting and maintaining health behaviors or recovery from illness which have physical, psychocultural, and social significance or meaning for those being assisted generally by a professional nurse or one with similar role competencies.[4]

Professional Nursing Care refers to those cognitive and culturally learned behaviors, techniques, processes, or patterns that enable (or help) an individual, family, or community to improve or maintain a favorable healthy condition or lifeway.[3]

IMPORTANCE OF CARE: SOME ASSUMPTIONS AND HYPOTHESES

A world of frequent change, violence, wars, and conflicts makes one realize that care is essential to help protect, develop, nurture, and provide survival to people in a variety of ways. The anthropologic record of the long survival of humans makes us pause to consider the role of care in the evolution of humankind. Different ecologic, cultural, social, and political contexts have influenced human health care and the survival of the human race. One can speculate that cultures could have destroyed themselves had not humanistic care acts helped to reduce intercultural stresses and conflicts and protect humans. Today, people vaguely know that care is vital to recovery from illness and to maintenance of healthy lifeways. From the human record, care attitudes and behavior have been important in the past, as they are today. A question to ponder is: What would the world be like today without human caring services? Some of these philosophic, historic, and cultural perspectives about the importance of care have been presented by the author in another publication.[3]

To consider further the importance of care, several major postulates and assumptions have been identified in the literature. They are as follows:

1. Human caring is a universal phenomenon, but the expressions, processes, and patterns of caring vary among cultures.

2. Caring acts and processes are essential for human birth, development, growth, and survival, and for a peaceful death.

3. Caring is the essence of and unifying intellectual and practical dimension of professional nursing.

4. Care has biophysical, cultural, psychologic, social, and environmental dimensions that must be explicated and verified to provide truly holistic care to people.

5. Nursing acts are transcultural and require nurses to identify and use intercultural nurse-client and system data.

6. Care behaviors, goals, and functions vary with social structure and specific values of people from different cultures.

7. Self and other care practices vary in different cultures and in different care systems.

8. The identification of universal and nonuniversal folk and professional caring behaviors, beliefs, and practices is essential to advancing the body of nursing and generic care knowledge.

9. Care is largely culturally derived and requires culturally based knowledge and skills for efficaciousness.

10. There can be no curing without caring, but there may be caring without curing.[3]

In addition, the following theoretic statements and hypotheses have been developed to stimulate further investigations about caring:

1. Intercultural differences in care beliefs, values, and practices reflect identifiable differences in nursing care practices.

2. Cultures that highly value individualism with independence modes will show signs of self-care practices and values; whereas cultures that do not value individualism with independence modes will show limited signs of self-care practices and more signs of other-care practices.

3. There is a close relationship between caregiver and care receiver behaviors.

4. People from different cultures can identify caring and noncaring behaviors and attitudes.

5. The greater the differences between folk care values and professional care values, the greater the signs of cultural conflict and stresses between professional caregivers and nonprofessional care receivers.

6. Technologic caring acts, techniques, and practices differ cross-culturally and have different outcomes for health and nursing care practices.

7. The greater the signs of dependency upon technology to give care, the greater the signs of depersonalized human care to clients.

8. Symbolic and ritual forms of nursing care behaviors have different meanings in different cultures, which necessitates knowledge of the meaning and functions of care symbols and rituals.

9. There is a close relationship between political, religious, economic, and cultural values and the quality of health care services rendered.[3]

Unquestionably, many more challenging hypotheses could be stated to help nurses realize the multiple areas in which care may be investigated.

There is a potential for nurses to develop a scientific and humanistic body of care knowledge with practice skills. Such a body of knowledge could become not only the distinctive and unique feature of the discipline of nursing, but could also be the major guide to nursing interventions and health maintenance. Transcultural *specific* and *universal care* knowledge is greatly needed to guide nursing decisions in caring for individuals, families, and communities. Such knowledge would be essentially new and would provide rich bases for guiding nursing education and practice. Knowledge of *all* cultures will someday be a major and powerful source supporting nursing principles and the laws that guide nurses' thoughts and actions. That day is in the distant future.

It is ironic that the word "care" has been commonly used by nurses for nearly a century, and yet the meaning, characteristics, processes, types, and divergent expressions of care have been only limitedly identified and validated.[2] Presently, there is only a small number of nurse researchers investigating care phenomena per se. The interest, however, is steadily growing, especially among graduate students and recent graduates of doctoral programs in nursing.

The cultural care movement began with the initiation of the Transcultural Nursing Care Conferences in 1973 and with National Research Caring Conferences in 1975.[3,6] As a consequence of these conferences, a core of nurse researchers began to focus on a systematic study of care concepts and practices. There was a heightened interest among nurse researchers to reexamine the nature, importance, and components of care, and to reflect upon why care has been neglected as an area of study. Several nurses said to the author, "We are glad you took the leadership to promote and advance the study of care, because it is not understood and valued in nursing—only in a vague way." Nurses did examine care anew as something they had taken for granted many years. Most assuredly, the national conferences and publications on care over the past decade have helped nurses reexamine care and investigate it systematically as a unique or special domain of nursing. Recently, nursing students have become avid learners about care, but they also remain baffled as to why nurses and the nursing profession have been so indifferent about or negligent in its study, teaching, and practice until recently.

Care studied from a transcultural nursing perspective has opened entirely new vistas of knowledge. The concepts of *care-specific* and *care-universal* have been entirely new and stimulating approaches for most nurses. Studying care from a cross-cultural view has been overwhelming to most nurses who have not been educated in transcultural nursing or who have no knowledge of anthropology. The author's transcultural studies of care have revealed that care values and behaviors differ within and between cultures.[4] There are diverse care values and patterns of giving care in different cultural and subcultural groups in the United States and in other places in the world. For example, the New Guinea people of Melanesia value surveillance and protection as essential care; whereas Southern rural Afro-Americans in the United States greatly value and practice concern and support as care.[7]

To date, the author has found that care behaviors, values, and expressions exist in all human cultures, but its characteristics and values tend to be different and largely covert. Care appears to be the hidden quality of human services that makes people satisfied or unsatisfied with health services. Care will require far more scrutiny than cure because of its subtle, hidden, and philosophically embedded attributes. Care phenomena are difficult to explicate, and we need different ways to study and verify care. We need qualitative and new methods to study care and health.[8]

Most important, care promises to be a truly special feature that will legitimize nursing as a professional and academic discipline. Many nurses are slow to envision this potential, however. Will nurses awaken to the importance of care after other disciplines make it known or "scientific?" I contend that nursing has a richer and longer historic claim to care phenomena than any academic or professional discipline. We must, however, diligently study, verify, and use knowledge about care with much more vigor than in the past. Care also remains a major way to legitimize nursing and make its unique contribution to humanity known to the public. No concept or line of research could be more important to nurses and the nursing profession than care. Will we meet this challenge?

CRITICAL ISSUES TO DISCOVERING CARE

In order to discover the essence and unique features of care, several issues and factors must be considered. The following factors need investigation in order to discover and understand care as the essence of nursing and health.

First, there is the central major issue related to whether or not nurses want to value care and have it as a central focus and unique domain of nursing. If nurses collectively do not value care and do not see it as important to nursing now and in the future, then care will not prevail as the essence of nursing. If nurses are not taught and socialized to know about and to use care in providing client services, then the concept will be strange and limitedly used by them. This is a critical problem today, since many nursing school faculty still seem to be focusing on medical diagnostic and treatment regimens, with only scantly interspersed mention of care in nursing theory, practice, and research. Several nursing students have repeatedly told the author, "Very few faculty teach us about care; instead we spend our time learning symptoms of disease conditions, cure treatment modes, and how to be a curer rather than a carer." What do faculty see as the heart of nursing? What are faculty teaching and practicing as care? Have medical cures for specific diseases taken too firm a hold on nursing students and faculty? What care content and experiences do nursing students learn about today in schools of nursing? Are nurse specialists practicing care or predominantly medical curing practices?

Linn's earlier study of the attitudes of nurses and physicians regarding care and cure revealed that medical faculty was more cure oriented than nursing faculty.[9] There were no statistically significant differences between the means of nursing students and the nursing faculty sampled. Her study revealed, however, that medical students tend to place more importance on patient cure than do nursing students. Perhaps there is still hope for reaffirming care as the essence and distinctive feature of nursing; however, from workshops held across the United States from 1978 to 1983, the author has found a generation of nursing students who say that they are not taught to know and practice care per se.[10] She has also observed and frequently heard older nurses express a nostalgic view of the past: "We used to practice care, but now we can't, due to demands upon our time to monitor machines, and deal with a whole new array of noncaring activities." These older nurses are encouraged to hear that care is being brought back into nursing and being rigorously studied.

Second, there is the issue related to ambiguities in the linguistic uses of the word "care." Gaut has documented that most nurses tend to use "care" as a slogan and a meaningless action to provide health services.[11] The author has frequently heard nurses say, "I give care," "I give personalized care to my patients," "I provided care to Mr. Jones." What does the concept of care mean to nurses and to clients? What are the intended or nonintended uses of the word by nurses? "Care" at times appears also to have magical and ritualistic attributes that are not clearly understood by clients and by nurses. Does the expression "I give personalized care" imply magical and ritualistic acts that are always beneficial to clients? Do nurses believe that beneficial care is implicit simply in the use of the word? In general, care remains an ambiguous and vague concept, but a term frequently used by nurses. Will nurses take the position of explicating the meaning and uses of the word "care?" How can nurses become knowledgeable about the meanings and explicit uses of care?

The *third* critical issue related to care is the diverse way that it is expressed by the actions of nurses and clients of different cultures in the world. There are marked cultural differences and some similarities in the way nurses give care and in the way clients expect it to be given. The author's study of thirty cultures clearly indicates that differences are more prevalent than universals.[4] Nonetheless, she holds that through systematic ethnographic and ethnocaring research, we will discover some universal aspects of care along with the differences. Universal features of care will be identifiable and will be related to actions that are directed at human survival and protection of humans under life-threatening conditions. *Diversity of care* will be more dominant due to marked differences in the social structure and cultural values of people. These postulates about universal and specific care have guided the author's research since the early 1960s, and to date many different nursing care behaviors have been identified. There are also care universals observed by nurses who give care in specific cultures. For example, Canadian nurses emphasize and practice supportive measures, whereas American nurses tend to use psychophysiologic stress alleviation as care.[4] Hospitals and clinics also vary in their values and norms related to care and cure emphases.

In general, nurses need to think about what is universal about care and what is culture-bound in their practices and beliefs. In so doing, similarities and differences in care will become known. What can help nurses shift their culture-bound or ethnocentric views about care to a worldwide or transcultural perspective? Will nurses be willing to study changes in values and practices over time? These questions and others make us realize the work that needs to be done to make care more overt than covert, and more central than diffused in research and in practice.

There is also the issue of whether nurses will be interested in studying the differences between *folk* and *professional* care practices. From transcultural nursing and anthropologic research, we know that there are differences between professional and folk caregivers and recipients of health care.[12] More and more cultures are able to identify the differences between their local or folk care practices and those of professional health providers. Some people find marked incongruities between folk values and professional care services, which pose serious problems in receiving or continuing with nursing and health care services. Most nurses need transcultural nursing knowledge to be able to identify differences and similarities between various practices. With only 150 to 300 nurses in the world prepared and qualified to be transcultural nursing specialists, researchers, teachers, and clinicians, the discovery of folk and professional knowledge will take some time. Transcultural nurses have been largely prepared in the United States and are working diligently to establish care and transcultural nursing as a subdiscipline. There is a need for more transcultural nurses to study all cultures and nursing care practices in the world. Hence, much work and planning ahead is needed in order to discover the rich and untapped knowledge about universal and nonuniversal care and nursing care phenomena.

The *fourth* critical issue related to care is whether nurses will begin to theorize about and verify therapeutic and nontherapeutic care practices. Hypodeductive and inductively based theories with concomitant research are needed to determine the efficacy of nursing care interventions. What is difficult to realize is that more than 100 years have elapsed since professional nursing was born, and still the nature, functions, and theories of specific care phenomena—ie, surveillance, comfort, presence, and others—have not undergone theoretic speculation or investigation, except by a few nurse researchers. Again, most nurses have been actively involved in focusing upon medical phenomena, ie, symptoms, diagnostic methods, and treatments. The medical and technologic revolution (post-World War II) forced nurses to give more attention to medical tasks than to care (such as empathy, sympathy, touch, compassion, love, trust, sharing, succor, nurture and other care constructs). To date, researchers have discovered nearly 50 care constructs in transcultural studies; some of them are unknown to nurses living in a particular culture.[4] These constructs need to be studied and verified to advance nursing *care* knowledge and to guide nursing care interventions. Are nurse researchers and theoreticians willing to focus on care phenomena in order to know the nature, essence, and practice of professional care?

A *fifth* issue closely related to the abovementioned one is the current trend among some nurses to be attracted to physicians' work as "medical curers" with dramatic cures, lucrative salaries, and public powerful images in society. Some nurse clinicians and faculty continue to be enamoured with technologic tools and biomedical treatment modes. The curative medical model with medicine's cultural values of being "all-knowing" about medical matters may be quite attractive to nurses. Rather than becoming excited about nursing care models and how care heals and helps clients to recover in significant ways, they may opt for curing. It is disconcerting to hear some nurses say, "I do not have time to care for clients by listening to them, or to provide support, comfort, and other caring acts" because of their responsibilities to physicians to do these medical tasks. Have nurses drifted unknowingly into the medical model and forsaken care as the essence or heart of nursing? Do nurses perceive cure as the heart of nursing? How can we help nurses learn to value and know care fully and to gain satisfaction through highly knowledgeable and competent skills of care? The critical issue is whether it is too late to redirect or resocialize nurses from medical curing and task practices to nursing care practices. If nurses are victims of medical technologies and medical cure ideologies, then the nursing profession faces major problems in socializing nurses to value and practice care. Care must become more a part of nurses' thinking and actions before a viable care culture can be legitimized and maintained. We need to find ways to resocialize nurses toward valuing care and to teach them care principles, processes, and intervention modes.

A *sixth* important issue of long standing is whether the nursing profession will take a *public* stand to declare *care* a *central, unifying, unique, and dominant feature and discipline-based knowledge of nursing as a profession.* Recently, and most encouragingly, the Canadian Nurses Association has adopted care as being central to nursing.[13] Will the American Nurses Association and other world nursing associations make care a dominant focus to guide nursing education and nursing practices? Currently, the American Academy of Nursing and other nursing organizations tend to be focused on public policies, building a positive public image, establishing autonomy, influencing politicians, and establishing professional unity and Centers for Nursing. One must ask: What efforts are being made to identify and verify the distinctive and unique components of nursing as a discipline and profession? Nurses could well make a significant forward thrust if its members were willing to establish nursing's unique, central, and major domains, such as the concept of care. Moreover, if care were supported as a major theoretic, philosophic, and historic component of nursing, one could predict that the above-mentioned activities would bring a positive image, better economic conditions, and public visibility to nursing.

It is often difficult for colleagues in other disciplines to understand why the nursing profession has not explicated or established its major boundaries to make it an academic discipline. For example, the discipline of anthropology focuses on the study of people through time and place. Sociologists focus on social interactions, families, and social systems. What is nursing's dominant thrust? I believe that care within a health and cultural context could be the distinct component that distinguishes nursing from other disciplines.

Currently, nurse theorists and some nursing leaders are emphasizing concepts such as man, health, environment, energy (wave frequencies), adaptation, stress, coping, perception, human responses, interpersonal relationships, and social systems to explain nursing.[14-18] While these theoretic constructs are important and do influence nursing, the author does not believe that they will ultimately be found to be central, distinct, unifying, or special boundary features of nursing as a profession and discipline. We know that many well-established disciplines such as anthropology, sociology, and physics have systematically studied and made claims to various phenomena, especially man, family, health, energy, systems, human responses, and environment. Theoreticians and researchers in these disciplines have acquired in-depth and expert knowledge about these phenomena. While any discipline may use and make claims to any knowledge, and knowledge has no fixed boundary, still there are norms and expectations regarding domains of knowledge. Scientists and humanists make claims to their knowledge domains by virtue of their research and in-depth experience on the subject. One must ask if nurse theorists and researchers have been sufficiently prepared in depth and breadth to master constructs of energy waves, environment, ecology, and other areas to use them knowingly in nursing and from a discipline perspective. Moreover, will the abovecited knowledge areas be adequately developed and reformulated to know and explain nursing in a meaningful and accurate way? This will not occur unless nurses become well prepared in the general and specific knowledge of these domains. Without such in-depth knowledge, it can be an exercise in futility, providing only superficial insights. While nurses may continue to use the constructs of environment, energy, families, systems, and human responses, the author predicts that they will not ultimately characterize nursing. She holds that care and health will far more commonly be used to explain and predict nursing by the year 2000.

Recently, the American Nurses Association published a social policy statement and defined nursing as "the diagnosis and treatment of human responses to actual or potential health problems."[19] The rationale for the selection of "human response" to characterize nursing and its epistemologic and philosophic dimensions are unknown and unexplained. Why "human response?" What makes this term unique or special to nursing? "Human responses" has certainly not been a unique domain of or traditionally used term in nursing. It appears to the author to be an attempt to establish a new term to describe nursing that has long been used and studied in other disciplines, especially psychology and anthropology. Moreover, it is more than human responses with which nurses are concerned. Hence, perceptive nurses are baffled about "human responses." Moreover, nurses question whether they have been prepared and qualified truly to know and understand human responses, especially with limited sociocultural and psychologic knowledge of human responses, and especially of different cultures. Perhaps "human responses" was selected as a term of political and social unity rather than as a substantive term to establish nursing's body of knowledge. Furthermore, the illustrations cited in the social policy statement—such as the focus for nursing interventions related to pain, impaired functions, dysfunctional perceptual orientations to health, and so forth—tend to be more a medical curative focus than nursing's traditional care, prevention, and health focus.[19]

Why have the creators of this policy statement eschewed or avoided the concept of care as the central and unique core of nursing? This latest cultural trend in nursing—to grasp some idea to attract nurses and to get political unity and public visibility—is fascinating. The author predicts that this latest catchword, "human response," will not directly move us forward and will only deter nurses from dealing with care as the essence of nursing. One can, of course, hope that it might make nurses realize the importance and value of care. Some nurses believe that health per se will be the distinctive domain of nursing, but we know that other health professions have laid claims to health for some time. It is now the linguistic and general framework for *all* the health professions, including nursing. Unquestionably, nursing has much to offer regarding health promotion and maintenance. The author predicts that it will remain a general framework for all professions, and that nursing's link to health will be related directly to care phenomena.

Of course, one would be remiss not to add briefly that care has undoubtedly been eschewed by some nurses because they see it as sex-linked with the feminine caregiver role. They might avoid using the term because they perceive it as a demeaning term with less social prestige than cure. However, now that males are learning and systematically discovering care and its constructs, such as love and support, some nurses are beginning to reevaluate care as being of considerable value. Because of past links with the concept and the women's role, however, it may take a while for nurses to overcome past cultural beliefs.

With the above-mentioned critical issues in mind, there is concern as to *how* and *when* nursing will establish itself as a knowledgeable and legitimate discipline and profession having its own distinct body of knowledge. Nursing as a discipline means that there is a cadre of scholars developing, testing, and refining domains of knowledge areas to support its raison d'etre. The domain(s) of knowledge should reflect the primary intellectual and practical features of nursing. Nurses are responsible for generating and transmitting such knowledge to their colleagues and the public. To date, there are 28 doctoral (PhD, ND, DNSc, and so forth) programs for nurses (and several more soon to be established).[20] The critical problem remains: Nursing's body of knowledge has been identified in a limited manner. It seems imperative, therefore, that nurses begin to identify, test, and verify nursing's unique knowledge domains systematically *as a discipline*. Students enrolled in nursing's highest degree program should have access to knowledge that makes nursing a discipline and a profession. Doctoral students should be challenged to build upon this knowledge, which in turn should help to justify and legitimize the existence of doctoral programs in nursing. Will nurses face this critical issue and consider care as one major and essential discipline awaiting discovery by nurse researchers? It has been interesting to find that the rationales offered for doctoral programs have generally not included *care* as the major distinguishing phenomenon of nursing.[21] This fact has often been baffling to other disciplines who perceive nurses as exquisite caregivers. The author has found that many academic disciplines are quick to envision the phenomenon of care as a basis for legitimizing doctoral programs for nursing in academic institutions, and are struck why nurse leaders avoid the concept and rely on borrowed concepts from the physical and social sciences.

Nursing is at a point in history where its leaders and followers must use knowledge that can guide nurses' thoughts, decisions, and actions. No longer can nurses continue to be expected to borrow on other disciplines' knowledge alone. We must make known and share nursing's knowledge with other disciplines. How can nurses best pursue, explicate, and verify the meaning and function of care within nursing, and from a transcultural perspective? This is a major challenge to nursing students, researchers, and theoreticians. Care could well be its essential and distinctive feature. One can predict that if nurses would focus on care to establish a body of knowledge, nursing could be fully recognized and valued as a viable profession and discipline. Most important, care should be studied from a scientific and humanistic perspective to delineate the true nature of nursing. The use of qualitative research will be important in discovering the humanistic and scientific aspects of care. Qualitative research provides data on the meanings, attributes, essences, and other understandable features of care to make it a meaningful concept for nurses and the public. Quantitative and qualitative research provides many avenues to understanding and documenting the focus of care.

In sum, care remains the essence of nursing. It is the unique, major, boundary feature of nursing, and one of its most promising areas of study. Knowledge about care is needed in society to help individuals, families, and community groups. Such knowledge is greatly needed today to establish nursing as a discipline and profession, and to improve or maintain health care services. Once care is examined in its fullest breadth and depth, then the author predicts that nursing's public image, economic worth, political posture, academic value, and other desired values and goals will become clearer. Nursing as a discipline will find its place in society and in academic institutions through the explication and use of care.

REFERENCES

1. Leininger M: Caring: The essence and central focus of nursing. Nurses Found (Nursing Research Report) 12(1):2, 14, 1977.
2. Leininger M: Caring: A central focus for nursing and health care services. Nursing Health Care 1(3):135–143, 176, 1980.
3. Leininger M: Caring: An Essential Human Need. Proceedings of the Three National Caring Conferences. Thorofare, NJ, Charles B. Slack, Inc, 1981.
4. Leininger M: Transcultural Nursing: Concepts, Theories and Practices. New York, John Wiley and Sons, 1978.
5. Webster's New World Dictionary of the American Language. Cleveland and New York, World Publishing Company, 1970, p 496.
6. Leininger M: Proceedings of the National Transcultural Nursing Conferences. New York, Masson International Publishing Company, 1979.
7. Leininger M: Ethnocaring, ethnohealth, and social structure of selected rural southern cultures. Funded study, summer, 1981.
8. Leininger M: Qualitative Research Methods in Nursing. New York, Grune & Stratton *(in press)*.
9. Linn LS: A survey of the "care-cure" attitudes of physicians, nurses, and their students. Nursing Forum 14:145–159, 1975.
10. Personal communication with nurses in the United States from 1978 to 1983.
11. Gaut DA: Conceptual analysis of caring: research method. *In* Caring: An Essential Human Need. Proceedings of the Three National Caring Conferences. Thorofare, NJ, Charles B. Slack, Inc., 1981, pp 17–24.
12. Leininger M: Transcultural nursing: Its progress and its future. Nursing Health Care 2(7):365–371, 1981.
13. Personal communication with Dr. Shirley Stinson, President of the Canadian Nurses Association, 1982.
14. Rogers ME: An introduction to the theoretical basis of nursing. Philadelphia, PA. F.A. Davis, 1970.
15. Riehl JP, Roy C (eds): Conceptual Models for Nursing Practice. New York, Appleton-Century-Crofts, 1974, pp 134–157.
16. King I: Toward a Theory for Nursing. New York, John Wiley and Sons, 1971.
17. Levine M: The four conservation principles in nursing. Nursing Outlook 21(3):171–175, March 1973.
18. Auger JR: Behavioral Systems and Nursing. Englewood Cliffs, NJ, Prentice-Hall, Inc., 1976.
19. American Nurses' Association (ANA). Nursing: A social policy statement. Kansas City, MO, December, 1981.
20. National League for Nursing (NLN). Doctoral programs in nursing 1982–83. New York, National League for Nursing, 1982.
21. Personal communication with faculties of several universities, in which the author served as a consultant to doctoral programs.

2

A Philosophic Orientation to Caring Research

There are three questions that offer some organization for thinking about philosophy and caring research:

1. What is philosophic orientation?

2. Why philosophy in science?

3. Why philosophy in nursing science?

I. PHILOSOPHIC ORIENTATION

What is a philosophic orientation or what does it mean to claim a philosophic orientation? Does one face the East or West as one ponders the great truths of life and ask questions like, "What is the nature of reality?", "What is the nature of knowledge?", or "What is the nature of value?" Perhaps a philosopher is a person who claims allegiance to a school of thought such as idealism, pragmatism, or realism, and thus is able to face the world with calmness and composure, knowing the appropriate questions to ask. Maybe, like Socrates, one would philosophize all the time.

The author does not pretend to have an answer to the proposed question. In addressing the subject of philosophy and caring research, she does not have a philosopher's stone whereby she might change the base metal of thought, but she does propose an activity. While the schools of philosophy do allow for the classification of human thought, the danger of such categorization lies in allowing the names of various classifications to become labels that are used as substitutes for thought rather than as tools for thinking. In view of such danger, it is perhaps less important to know the subject of philosophy as it is to learn to philosophize.

Plato said, "Thought is a dialogue and we are all members of a society of potential thinkers." The author's orientation is toward recognizing the potential for a shared dialogue—a collective consciousness of human beings using language to inquire and talk to each other. "Orientation" in one sense refers to a homing faculty of certain animals. We seem to be animals exceptionally good at thinking. Using language, the unique gift of nature, we are exploring and becoming a network of thought as we measure things, turn things over, and attempt to discover the meaning of caring in its fullest dimensions.[1]

We make language together and are bound together by speech. Our shared interest in nursing and caring links us together in a common mind attempting to explore the truth of caring. The author would suggest that philosophy will provide a framework and direction for thinking about caring, which might otherwise meander indefinitely among the vast plains of our collective intellects.

Philosophy springs from the need to organize ideas and find meaning in thoughts and actions. In search of meaning, one would direct philosophic thought and inquiry in three directions:

1. The contemplative or speculative, considered to be the traditional approach to questions about the "whole of reality."

2. The prescriptive or normative, which recommends values and ideals. The "ought" statements are derived from the evaluation of facts.

3. Criticism or analysis, which is concerned with the clarification of concepts and propositions, and attempts to answer questions about the meaning of terms and expressions while also examining the logical relations and presuppositions that the terms and expressions involve.[2]

Because the central purpose of this chapter is to explore and examine concepts, meanings, functions, and relationships embedded within the construct of caring, the commentary is limited to the third aspect of philosophic inquiry, analysis. In this approach, the analyst is concerned with clarifying the arguments and methods employed by human beings in their speech and thought, and with formulating criteria for adequate theorizing.

With this introduction, we proceed to the second question posed—Why philosophy in science? The linkages between science and analytic philosophy are discussed first.

II. ANALYTIC PHILOSOPHY AND SCIENCE

There are different senses of the word "science" used by scholars today. In one sense, "science" is used to designate an a priori set of absolute judgments arranged to hang together in a formal system. In another sense, there is science in the world around us—a complex of changing concepts whose only reality is that the concepts give order to and are tested by the empiric facts.

The etymologic origin of "science" refers to broad theoretic inquiry. Dewey in his early work on the philosophy of science urged, "We must take the idea of science with some latitude. . .with sufficient looseness. Science signifies the existence of systematic methods of inquiry, which when brought to bear on a range of facts enables us to understand them better and control them more intelligently."[3]

The word "science" is not to be confused with the term "scientific method." Unlike science, the scientific method is not a way of thinking or an attitude, but a procedure for working out a problem. It is how the problem is conceived and justified as being significant that involves matters of choice and value judgments; and it is in the stages of problem definition and justification that the essential philosophic questions must be asked.

Science, like philosophy, is an activity—the activity of arranging the known facts in groups under general concepts and then judging the concepts by the factual outcomes of the actions that we base on them. The activity of science is directed at one end—finding the material truth. While the findings of science are neutral, as every fact and grouping of facts is neutral, the activity of science, which finds the facts and orders them, is not neutral.[4]

Stephen Gould, a leading evolutionary biologist, commented in a recent interview on how science changes with the political climate. He noted that: "The rise and fall in popularity of scientific theories correlates with changes in the political and social climate."[5] This is not a new observation, but one that needs repeating. Science does not stand apart from other human institutions just because its methodology leads to objective knowledge. Rather, science might be considered to be embedded in society, and scientists reflect the social prejudices of their own lives, classes, and culture. Because of this, Gould suggests there is a desperate need for scientists to scrutinize more rigidly the sources of justification for their beliefs.

At a recent conference on science and human values, the participants warned of the tunnel-vision approach of science and technology and its imminent threat to humanism.[6] It would seem that such an assumption could only occur from semantic confusion, wherein we equivocate the words "science" and "technology" and turn the word "science" into a distinct specialization. With such confusion, assumptions are often made that science is necessarily about only quantifiable things, and that any academic subject with the word "science" in it is therefore scientific. Terms such as "statistical significance" or "cognitive process research" become part of the "scientific" language that somehow assures value free and legitimate science.

A good example of confusion can be found in the discussion of why the social sciences, including nursing, are radically different from other sciences. The claim is made that social sciences differ because they require a methodology radically unlike that required in the other sciences. If we examine this claim, it will become apparent that there is confusion between "methodology" and "technique," in much the same way that the words "science" and "technology" are confused.

One point needs to be clarified. To assert that techniques differ between disciplines is not a drastic claim, and, indeed, it is one that could easily be substantiated. Given that technology refers to the techniques and materials used to achieve the objectives of science, it is easy to justify that experimental control is perhaps more applicable to the phenomenon of physics than to the phenomenon of nursing. Accepting such a claim of differing techniques, however, does not allow for the radical claim that there is a significant difference between disciplines because of methodology.

Such a claim would require that nursing demand a different methodology—a different logic of inquiry—than physics. To hold such a view is to deny that all of science is characterized by a common methodology, a common logic of justification applied to its acceptance or rejection of hypotheses of theories. There is a context in which nursing as a social science is methodologically distinguished from the other sciences, but that distinction does not substantiate the claim of significant difference between disciplines.

A logical methodology of validation, explanation, or prediction is precisely what is referred to when it is asserted that the scientific method is pervasive through all the sciences. The methodology of science is applicable to the investigation of social as well as nonsocial phenomena.[7]

Maslow reminds us that the first obligation of science is to confront all of reality as human beings experience it—to describe, understand, and accept all of it, and not to deny reality or refuse to confront aspects of it because they are not amenable to study with the best instruments at hand. Researchers who restrict themselves to doing only that which they can do elegantly with the techniques already available tend to define science as that which they are able to do. That which they are not able to do becomes "nonscience" or unscientific.[8] However, the researchers who choose to work as best they can with important problems invent new ways of defining science.

This "problem-centering" approach allows for philosophy and seeks it as a source of science, knowing that it provides working hypotheses of comprehensive application. The hypotheses serve as working ideas and provide a wider, more general view. Without such a view, special investigation becomes barren and one-sided. This is especially true in the early formative stages of a new science such as nursing. Let us now consider exactly what philosophy has to offer science.

III. RELATIONSHIP BETWEEN PHILOSOPHY AND SCIENCE

There is a reciprocal relationship between philosophy and science, each feeding upon the other, and yet each maintaining definite distinctions. Consider that in every discipline or subject, there is a serial progression from the specific to the more general. Science lies closer to the specific pole and philosophy closer to the general, but there is no definite line where one ends and the other begins. Ideas originating at the philosophic end (general, vague, speculative) have been indispensable factors in the generation of science, for these ideas are then tested and modified as they suggest and direct the detailed work of science. Ideas originating from philosophic questions provide the more whole, general view so necessary to science. Philosophy becomes a source of science in the degree to which it provides working hypotheses of comprehensive application, which can be tested and modified as they are used in directing the detailed work of observation and understanding.[3]

IV. ANALYTIC PHILOSOPHY

The task widely assumed to be distinctive to philosophy has been to assess and systematically relate the diversity of human knowledge and experience from an integrating perspective. Philosophy is a fundamental science because it is the most general science of existence. Its major objective is to discover the basic kinds and structures of reality, and to establish the necessary principles that constitute the intellectual foundations of knowledge of all specialized subject matter. This conception of the aim of philosophy does not suppose that philosophy can supply the foundational principles, the moral, or the definitive procedures for certifying propositions about human knowledge, action, or values. It does assume that there is a class of questions that arises in connection with every specialized subject which is generally regarded as being characteristically philosophic because the questions deal with foundational problems of knowledge.[9]

Examples of foundational problems include clarifying such notions as "growth" or "adaptation" in biology, "instinct" or "purpose" in psychology, "democracy" or "property" in political science, "responsibility" or "self-development" in moral theory, and "caring" or "therapeutic use of self" in nursing.

The task of philosophy, then, is to critique cognitive claims and make the researcher self-conscious about the nature and grounds of intellectual commitments, and to enlarge further one's angle of vision by suggesting alternative ways of organizing portions of thought. We are addressing philosophic questions when we ask under what general conditions discourse is meaningful, when we examine the grounds of belief dominating an area of inquiry, when we examine the logic implicit in evaluating the worth of evidence, or when we question the relationship of one branch of knowledge to some other branch.

Philosophy resembles the sciences in its exclusive appeal to rational argument and evidence. It is more general than science, however, for it not only tries to understand the world through science, but also attempts to comprehend science itself as a mode of understanding. Philosophers have tended to seek general perspectives by analysis of the roots—the basic concepts, assumptions, arguments, and inferences—characteristic of different domains. Although the procedures and standards of analysis vary considerably, as a basic task philosophers need to develop a system for the logical evaluation of their assertions—that is, the examination of ideas from the standpoint of clarity and the examination of arguments from the standpoint of validity.[10]

The philosophy of science is an integrating discipline. It articulates, assesses, and thereby helps to reorganize that logic of our knowledge, and the logical principles employed in establishing cognitive claims. The philosophy of science deals with problems emerging chiefly from those logically related sets of statements that constitute the theories of science. The main focus of attention becomes the linguistic aspects of the scientific enterprise.[7]

Philosophy, then, is an analysis of language, not of facts. The analysis of concepts is a coherent technique of thought which can be applied widely. It provides a specialized and appropriate method that can be used in answering many of the important and interesting questions that can be asked. Conceptual understanding is required, of course, in many contexts, but the technique of conceptual analysis gives a framework and direction to thinking about general questions and abstract concepts.[11] Nursing as a newly developing discipline requires just such a framework for its thinking and theory development. Let us move on to consider the third question: Why philosophy in nursing science?

V. PHILOSOPHY AND NURSING

To call for the application of philosophic methods to nursing is not to present a panacea for the practical difficulties attending nursing. Rather, it aims to improve our understanding of nursing by clarifying our conceptual apparatus—the ways in which we formulate beliefs, arguments, assumptions, and judgments concerning such topics as caring, support, motivation, and health.

Serious interest in nursing concepts and issues may be fused with serious concern for philosophic clarity and rigor. The basic significance of philosophic activity is rational reflection, critical analysis of arguments and assumptions, and systematic clarification of fundamental ideas. In applying philosophic methods of analysis, we are concerned directly with solving intellectual rather than practical problems, with removing the perplexities that arise in our attempt to say systematically and clearly what we are doing in nursing and why.

The need for philosophy in nursing was expressed by Crowley and Donaldson when they wrote:

> What is needed is the thinking of nurse philosophers and some philosophizing by nurse researchers. . .more explicit identification of what we are about in nursing research is imperative if we are to function truly as nurse researchers rather than as nurses conducting research in other disciplines.[12]

The problem lies not in devising the structure of the discipline of nursing, but in making the structure—that is, the broad conceptualizations and syntax of the discipline of nursing—explicit. Philosophic and similar types of enquiry within the discipline of nursing are crucial, not only for providing the knowledge base for professional preparation, but also for developing the discipline.

Nursing science has no history of relatively tested, solid, general principles or laws on which to fall back, like those of physics, chemistry, or biology. It is the tentative state of nursing science that renders it especially in need of direction by means of large and fruitful hypotheses. It is worth repeating that philosophy is a source of science in the degree to which it provides hypotheses. No matter how these are obtained, they are intrinsically philosophic in nature—good or bad philosophy, as the case may be. To treat them as scientific rather than philosophic is to conceal their hypothetical character and to freeze them into rigid dogmas that hamper, instead of assist, actual enquiry. What philosophy can contribute to nursing science is range, freedom, and constructive or creative invention. A researcher in any field gets preoccupied with more immediate urgencies and results, but when one begins to extend the range and the scope of thought, to consider obscure collateral consequences, then one begins to philosophize. Anyone is philosophic who makes a consistent effort to see and think in a more extensive time-span, or in reference to an enduring development as a whole.

The prestige of measurements in physical science should not be permitted to blind us to a fundamental question: To what extent is nursing a matter of forming specific skills and acquiring special bodies of information that are capable of isolated treatment? Exact quantitative determinations fall radically short of meeting the demands of interpersonal relationships, for they presuppose repetitions and exact uniformities.

Researchers may seek answers or questions outside nursing in material that already has scientific prestige, but such seeking is an abdication, a surrender. In the end it only lessens the chances that nursing, in actual operation, will provide the materials for an improved science. Nursing by its nature is an activity that includes science within itself. In its very process it identifies problems to be further studied, thus demanding more thought, more questions, and more science.

The sources of nursing science are any portions of knowledge that enter into the heart, head, and hands of nurses, and which by entering, make the performance of the nursing function more enlightened, more human, and more truly nursing. The discovery of nursing as science is never made; it is always in the making.

Nursing knowledge will be developed from nursing's unique perspective. By asking questions and viewing phenomena unlike those of other disciplines, nursing will develop a perspective from the practical fields of human environments and health. Nursing's perspective will further be defined by the phenomena it chooses to study and by its purpose for studying those phenomena. As Leininger wrote: "The way to understand nursing is to identify, describe, and research those central humanistic-scientific factors that are essential to effecting positive health change. . .the science of caring combines sciences with the humanities."[13]

Readers of this book have joined in an essential task facing nursing today: to clarify and make more explicit the unique perspective of and focus on nursing and caring. By defining caring as the phenomenon nurses choose to study, we as a group are in essence defining nursing's perspective. A word of caution is in order, however. If we state that caring is the essence of nursing, it is nursing that must incorporate a deeply human view of caring, and not caring which must be modified to fit the contemporary view of nursing. A review of the book's objective reassures us that our task of discovering caring in its fullest dimension is enlightened by philosophic questions and approaches.

CONCLUSION

At the beginning of this chapter, the author referred to nurses' being bound together by speech, making language become a live network of thought. Maybe everything we think is part of a cosmic network, and we are a kind of "caring consciousness" for the whole system. If the notion of a cosmic consciousness is untenable, perhaps there is a collective consciousness of human beings concerned about nursing and caring and other human beings. Consider not only the dimensions of caring, but also the dimensions of philosophic thought.

The world of creative philosophizing calls for three specific ways of thinking: (1) *Comprehensiveness of outlook*, which calls for a wholeness of vision; it is an invitation to "see life steadily and see it whole." (2) *Penetration*, which is a way of thinking that requires one to go beyond the usual slogans, the cliches, and the stereotypes, and demands that one dig to the roots of questions or problems to discover fundamental difficulties. (3) *Flexibility*, which is a call to be creative in thinking, to be nonjudgmental. All things are considered possible. Ask not, "What is it?" but ask, "What could it be?" Flexibility in research calls for tentative appraisals, hypothesis reappraisal, and reconstruction of judgment and action.

The aim of philosophic analysis is to clarify our thinking about science and about nursing by examining the logical features of the expressions and the arguments by which this thinking manifests itself. Faulty communication exacerbates disputes and diverts attention from the genuine issues. We become divided by the very language with which we seek to communicate. If we are to understand the problems, policies, and concepts of nursing, we would do well first to examine carefully the language of nursing discourse. We must respect the informal logic of words and expressions; when we know the true possibilities of language, we shall begin to communicate effectively. Effective communication will not guarantee mutual agreement, but it does guarantee mutual understanding.

In closing, the author would like to propose a few questions for pondering:

1. What are the means by which the caring function of nursing in all its phases can be conducted with a systematic increase in intelligent control and understanding?

2. What are the materials upon which we may and should draw in order to reduce the degree to which caring nursing activities are products of routine, tradition, and accidental influences?

3. From what sources shall we draw so that there shall be steady and cumulative growth of intelligent, communicable insight and direction in the understanding and researching of caring phenomena?

Nursing has the potential strength and leverage to help realign many of the prevailing distorted values in our society, but first we have to stop abandoning our values as women and nurses. Our task to bring about change is difficult because the questions nursing needs to ask are not the usual and more acceptable questions. Nursing needs detailed research in order to generate the essential questions and researchers who are sensitive to questions of value and "humanness" and caring. Although we desperately need theory and research, we also desperately need caring and human kindness.

REFERENCES
1. Thomas L: The strangeness of nature. N Eng J Med 298:1454, 1978.
2. Kneller G: Logic and Language of Education. New York, John Wiley and Sons, 1966, p 208.
3. Dewey J: The Sources of a Science or Education. New York, Liveright, 1929, pp 8, 51.
4. Boronowski J: The values of science. *In* Maslow AH (ed): New Knowledge in Human Values. Chicago, IL, H. Regnery Co., 1970, p 52.
5. Gould SS: How science changes with the political climate. US News and World Report 62, March 1, 1982.
6. Baum J: Science vs. humanities: the legacy of CP Snow. Change 3:11–13, 1981.
7. Rudner RS: Philosophy of Social Science. Englewood Cliffs, NJ, Prentice-Hall, 1966.
8. Maslow AH: The Psychology of Science. Chicago, IL, H. Regnery Co., 1966, p 16.
9. Nagel E: Philosophy in educational research. Phi Delta Kappa Symposium on Education Research, Bloomington, IN, 1960.
10. Scheffler I: The Language of Education. Springfield, IL, Charles C Thomas, 1974, p 5.
11. Wilson J: Thinking with Concepts. London, Cambridge University Press, 1963.
12. Donaldson SK, Crowley DM: Discipline of nursing: structure and relationship to practice. Communicating Nursing Research 10(9):1–21, 1977.
13. Leininger M: Preface. *In* Watson J (ed): Nursing: The Philosophy and Science of Caring. Boston, MA, Little, Brown & Co., 1979, p xii.

3

A Theoretic Description of Caring as Action*

A review of the nursing literature validated two major assumptions regarding the very special place of caring in nursing discourse:

1. Nursing heritage and traditions are firmly rooted in the value of care.

2. Caring is envisioned as a crucial and vital component of nursing.

The literature review highlighted one other aspect of caring that was the basis for this study: Although there were many statements in the literature that included the terms "care/caring," little attempt was made to clarify or explicate the terms.

"When I use a word," Humpty Dumpty said in a rather scornful tone, "it means just what I choose it to mean—neither more nor less." Humpty Dumpty, a master of words, knew that the stipulated definition is one that is given by the speaker, who asks that the defined terms consistently carry his meaning. This type of definition is frequently used as a matter of convenience, but such a definition could not be fairly justified or rejected by consideration of nonambiguous criteria.

At a time when the nursing profession is attempting to develop its own body of knowledge as an academic discipline, it becomes imperative that the language used to define theoretic concepts be precise, unambiguous, readily communicated, and justifiable. Concern for clarifying the use of "caring" in nursing discourse—and other conceptual questions—led to the methodology of concept analysis found in educational philosophy.

The goal of this study is to develop a strong theoretic description of caring that might lay the conceptual groundwork for further studies of caring. This study also attempts to show that in addition to the empiric questions that most often

*Paper presented at the Fourth National Caring Conference. Georgia Southern College, Statesboro, Georgia, March 18-20, 1981.

receive the attention of researchers, there are other kinds of questions and problems that require consideration if we are to understand and improve such practical enterprises as nursing. Caring is an example of such a conceptual problem, and its treatment here is intended to point out that an adequate theoretic description of caring is required before one can deal with the questions about caring competency that arise out of nursing practice.

In this chapter, the analysis of caring and related discussion are presented in the following format:

    I. Review of the purpose, specific aims, and background.

    II. Methodology.

    III. Logical conditions for use of the term "caring."

    IV. Action description based on logical conditions.

    V. Competency model of caring.

I. PURPOSE, AIMS, AND BACKGROUND

Purpose of Study

The purpose of this study is to clarify the concept "caring" by adequately describing the concept theoretically. The goal is to aid nurse educators and researchers in their use of the concept of caring. The theoretic description of caring is developed in terms of action categories that could be used to identify caring competencies and lay the conceptual groundwork for further studies.

Specific Aims

The specific objectives of this study are: (1) to address a set of questions utilizing the techniques of philosophic analysis; (2) to formulate a theoretic description of caring that is adequate to the task of identifying caring competencies; (3) to offer a systematic theoretic construction to which one can appeal in order to answer questions about how one improves a practical activity such as caring; (4) to propose a theoretic model of caring as action that has passed minimal tests of descriptive adequacy; that is, a description general enough to cover all cases or instances of caring, and yet specific enough to distinguish between any two cases of caring.

Background

Review of selected writings from philosophers, behavioral scientists, and nurses highlighted three points: (1) the importance of the notion of caring, as evidenced by the increasing frequency of the use of the concept; (2) the evolution of the concept of caring as related to other concepts; and (3) the discussion of activities such as feeding, touching, and talking, which, when grouped together, constituted caring.

The work of these scholars related caring directly and necessarily not only to the survival of the species, but also to the development of adult human beings capable of caring for and caring about others.[1-5]

Research studies in psychiatry and psychology emphasize the curative power of warm and caring relationships with clients.[6,7] In education, researchers found that the warmth and caring of teachers significantly increased learner achievement and adjustment in both primary grade and college level students.[8,9]

In response to the question, "Does caring make a significant difference in the health/illness experience of humans?" a growing body of evidence shows that the nurse's effect on the patient's welfare is greatly influenced by the relationship established and maintained with the patient.[10-12] The patient's perception of the caring relationship has also been studied, with the greatest number of responses indicating that person-to-person communication was especially indicative of caring behavior.[13]

Prior to 1975, there had been limited interest in the systematic study of the nature and essence of caring as a basis for nursing theory and practices. To quote Leininger: "The construct of care and caring is one of the most neglected yet important areas of study. Indeed caring from philosophic, linguistic, cultural, and professional viewpoints, has barely been studied with its variant forms of expressions and meaning."[14]

Part of the problem involved in thinking and talking about "caring" is the variety of the word's uses. In the nursing literature, for example, "caring" has no standard usage, and demands are placed upon the person using the term to clarify its sense, especially in discussions related to nursing education or nursing research. Confronted with such a problem, the author posed the following questions:

How might the concept of caring be rendered more meaningful for nursing discussions and nursing research?

How do we in nursing justify the use of the concept of "caring" in our discussions, teaching, and research? If caring is an idea central to the tasks of nursing, how is that idea taught?

Is the meaning of the concept of caring in the scholarly literature equivalent to the normal usage of the word? Have the scholars rendered the term more precise than in the common usage? Is the use of the concept of caring found in the nursing literature similar to the common usage and the related literature?

The conclusions reached from consideration of these questions included the following:

1. There is no clear-cut rule for the use of "caring" in common language, but the family of meanings is related to the notion of caring in three senses: (a) attention to or concern about; (b) responsibility for or providing for; and (c) regard or fondness for.

2. The meanings in the scholarly literature are equivalent to any one or more of the three senses of caring in common usage.

3. With the exception of Mayeroff, the nonnursing literature does not make the concept of caring more precise.[15]

4. The term "caring" in both lay and scholarly literature is found in discussions of: (a) certain feelings or dispositions within a person; (b) the doing of certain activities that seem to identify that person as a caring individual; or (c) a combination of both attitudes and actions in which caring about the other disposes the one to carry out activities for the other.

5. As a word, "caring" does not have one determinate definition and a singular meaning in all contexts; rather, it has a family of meanings, and its meaning shifts across contexts. It is the type of word that could be considered both vague and ambiguous.

The goal of this research was to develop a strong theoretic description of caring that would serve as conceptual groundwork for further studies. The varying uses of caring, however, render the term both vague and ambiguous. The search for precision and clarification of the term led the author to the analytic, linguistic approach found in educational philosophy.

II. PHILOSOPHY AS ANALYSIS

Philosophy aims explicitly at improving one's understanding of education and other important human endeavors, such as nursing, by the clarification of concepts. While philosophy is not an empiric enterprise, it can make research more successful by clarifying the concepts used in empiric research.[16]

Educational research can address two distinguishable sets of problems: (1) empiric, which, generally speaking, deals with matters of fact; and (2) philosophic, which deals in part with conceptual issues related to the process and discipline of education. The empiric researcher may ask questions that invite conceptual clarification or judgments that require justification. The difference between an empiric question and a conceptual one was noted by R.S. Peters:

> A scientific question is one that can in principle be answered by certain kinds of procedures in which observation and experiment play a crucial part. But the clarification and discussion of the concepts used and how they have meaning, and of the procedures by means of which these questions are answered, is a philosophical inquiry.[17]

Analysts are concerned with clarifying the arguments and methods employed by human beings in their speech and thought. The analytic approach uses second-order question (metaquestions) that require analysis of the terms themselves. The conceptual questions asked in that approach pertain to linguistic or logical relationships.

The aim of philosophic analysis is to clarify or systematize the language in which we express our scientific theories as well as our common-sense beliefs. [17,18] The aim of this analysis is to arrive at a description of caring that is both theoretically and conceptually adequate for a discussion of competency of caring in nursing.

There are several ways to approach the development of a theoretic description of caring. One might make a list of caring competencies or outline the criteria for doing so. Alternatively, one might list behaviors that seem to be perceived as caring by the one being cared for.

A description of caring derived from an arbitrary or stipulated set of criteria, however, is theoretic in its weaker sense. In its stronger sense, a theoretic description not only would include the constituents of caring and the relationship between the constituents, but also would meet certain tests of adequacy based on nonarbitrary criteria.[19]

These requirements incorporate certain guidelines for the development of a theoretic description of caring: (1) a formal or systematic approach to the consideration of the components or categories of caring; (2) identification of the relationship among the components of caring; and (3) adherence to certain criteria that would apply in the justification of the findings.

The word "description" rather than "definition" is used. Analytic philosophy attempts to formulate precisely the meanings of terms through techniques of explication rather than definition in its usual sense. Through explication, one studies the meaning of a term by studying its uses, and arrives at what might be called an "extended definition" or description of the term.[20]

The task of justifying a description of caring to be theoretically adequate would entail addressing at least three questions: (1) Did the analysis begin with "prior usage" consideration? (2) Does the description include the constituents of caring and the relationship among the constituents, and were these constituents logically and systematically considered? (3) Does the description of caring pass the test of descriptive adequacy in that it is general enough to cover all cases or instances of caring and specific enough to distinguish between any two cases of caring?

The description of caring sought in this study involved semantic analysis to focus on the use of the word in ordinary language, and explicative analysis to refine the term and render it unambiguous and theoretically adequate.

An explanation of the methodology follows.

III. METHODOLOGY FOR DEVELOPMENT OF AN ACTION DESCRIPTION OF CARING

The first step in developing a theoretic description of caring that could be justified by the criteria just listed is to address a set of questions that might serve as a logical framework for the discussion.

1. "How is the word 'caring' employed in normal usage, or why does one use the word 'caring' in this situation, and not in that?" (A caring/noncaring distinction)

2. "What logical conditions must be met to call any action a caring action; or, put another way; what must be true to say that S is caring for X?" (Action description)

The questions being asked in this analysis initially had to do with the predefinitional or ordinary usage of the word "caring," and with a consideration of the term "caring" as intentional human activity. Ordinary usage refers to the way in which a word or expression is regularly used, as opposed to nonstandard uses such as metaphysical, poetic, hyperbolic, extended, or deliberately restricted ones. The normal usage of a word serves as a nonarbitrary criterion for the development of conditions necessary for its employment.

In analyzing a practical activity like caring, the aim is not to invent a new concept or idea of caring, or even to specify what people ought to mean by caring. Rather, the objective is to study, clarify, and more thoroughly understand the idea of caring we already have.

Because caring is a practical activity, the question of what people do when caring is appropriate. When considering what people do, however, the "what" may be talked about in two very different ways—as sets of acts or as a set of actions. The distinction between act and action underlies the difference between a behavioral description and an action description of caring.

Act/Action Distinction

Kaplan, discussing explanation in behavioral science, specified two different ways to talk about "what people do"—as a set of acts or as actions. He explained:

> We may talk about it (the "what" people do) as a set of acts— biophysical operations, movements, or events; or we may talk about it as a set of actions—the acts in the perspectives of the actors, expressing certain attitudes and expectations, and thereby having a certain social and psychological significance.

> To arrive at an "act meaning," the scientist must construe what conduct a particular piece of behavior represents; to arrive at an "action meaning, " a search is made for the meaning of the interpreted action, its interconnections with other actions or circumstances.[21]

The author's concern with the concept of caring in nursing and the related issues of competency in and teaching of caring required her to give full attention to caring as a purposeful human activity, requiring an action description. While it might be possible to explain caring as a set of acts or behavior, her interest in further questions of competency and teachability necessarily involved a discussion of caring as an intentional human activity.

To assure the theoretic adequacy of the description, the following criteria were established:

1. An action description of caring rather than a behavioral description.

2. A description of caring that passed tests of conceptual adequacy.

3. A description of caring that could be justified as being theoretically adequate.

4. A description based upon common word usage rather than any technical or stipulated usage.

Addressing the term in its appropriate form and asking the question, "What must be true to say that S is caring for X?" the logical conditions necessary and sufficient to employ the concept were identified.

IV. LOGICAL CONDITIONS FOR CARING

The analysis of caring at this point distinguished between S caring or not caring for an object (X) in the sense of "providing for." Caring was considered an action one engages in or is occupied in doing, and as such the action is directed toward a goal. For the sake of precision and objectivity, the analysis considered S caring for an object rather than for a person. The discussion then extended to the consideration of S caring for self or other persons for the purpose of identifying what feature or features distinguish caring for persons from caring for objects.

It was determined that one might say that S is caring for X if and only if the following five conditions obtain:

1. S must be aware of the need for care in X (awareness).

2. S must know that certain things could be done to improve the situation (knowledge).

3. S must intend to do something for X (intention).

4. S must choose an action intended to serve as a means for bringing about a positive change in X, and must implement the action (+ change).

5. The positive change in X must be judged on the basis of what is good for X rather than for S or some other Y or Z (criterion welfare of X).

To refine the analysis even more and extend the consideration of caring for persons, the following questions were addressed:

1. In what sense must S be aware of X in order to care for X?

2. What must S know in order to care for X?

3. What is the relationship between the intended action, and the need for care?

The first condition for caring—awareness—calls for the ability to be aware of or to focus attention on X, whether X be an object or a person. However, caring for a person rather than an object requires a certain attitude in S. The attitude must be one of personal respect, that is, the kind of respect shown a person with human dignity. Such respect for other persons begins with regard for oneself as a human being worthy of personal respect, and is a necessary condition for all rational action among reasonable persons. To be able to say that S is caring for X, then S must be aware that that person has rights, dignity, and individual claims that demand respect.

The ability of S to identify the needs of X involves more than just awareness; it also involves various kinds of knowing. What must S know, however, in order to care for X? The knowledge involved in caring includes understanding the other's needs, knowing how to respond to those needs, and knowing one's own powers and limitations.[15] To consider S caring for X requires not only that S be aware of X and have enough knowledge about X to identify a need for care, but also, once a need is identified, knowing "what" to do about it in the sense of knowing that certain actions might improve the situation.

If one wishes to speak of S caring for X, it is not enough to say that S has identified a need for care and knows what to do; S also chooses to do something. The question then becomes, "What is the relationship between the intended action and the need for care?" Caring activity is intentional activity. One approach to the discussion of intention is to ask the questions: "What are you doing?" and "Why are you doing that?" The first question asks for a response in terms of the purpose or aim of the activity; the second question asks for a reason to justify such activity. Before qualifying an activity as caring or noncaring, one must first identify the intentions of S in terms of the purpose or aim of the activity, rather than basing one's judgment only on the observation of the activities of S.

To be considered to be caring, S must not only choose an action to meet a need for care in X, but must also intend the action to be a means of bringing about a positive change in X. At the very least, S should not intend injurious or hurtful activities. The implementation of any action, then, must be intended to serve as a means for bringing about a positive change in X. This brings us to the last question: "What would count as a positive change direction for X?"

In order to determine what would count as a positive change for X, one must be generally informed about the criteria according to which something would be accepted as good for all Xs as distinguished from Ys or Zs. What is good food for the lawn is not necessarily good for the car. What is good food for an 11-month-old infant is not necessarily good for either the lawn or the car. The notion of providing food as a means for positive change appears to be quite reasonable, but the judgment of whether the intended action is actually a means of bringing about a positive change would be based on what is good for the lawn (X), the car (Y), or the infant (Z).

One other distinction needs to be made. That is the distinction of what is good for this particular X, in this specific situation. Consider the example of a mother caring for her twin sons, aged 10 months. She has chosen to introduce solid foods into their feeding schedules to meet their needs for adequate nutrition. Given the conditions, could we say that the mother was caring? She identified the need for care (adequate nutrition), chose an action that she intended as the means to achieve a positive change (feeding solid foods to promote growth) based upon her knowledge about feeding children, and implemented the action by feeding the infants eggs and fruit twice a day. Based upon general knowledge about 10-month-old infants, one might say that this mother is caring. However, consider that infant A has an allergy to eggs: the mother is aware of that fact, but chooses to feed both children the same foods to save her time. Clearly she is not caring for infant A, because although in general, solid foods, especially eggs, are considered good for 10-month-old infants, this particular infant A has a need to avoid them. The judgment as to whether the intended action is a means for bringing about a positive change must be based on what is good for infant A, rather than infant B, or all other infants. The welfare-of-X criterion not only pertains to what is good for all infants in general, but also must include what is good for this particular infant according to its nature and specific circumstances.

The welfare-of-X consideration then becomes a nonarbitrary criterion which serves as a norm, standard, or principle for any activity intended or implemented as "means for positive change in X." The positive change would be judged solely on the criteria identified as being good for the welfare-of-X, thus excluding actions based on the whim or wishes of S or some other agent.

With these considerations in mind, the five conditions were refined and collapsed into three:

Condition I: S must have knowledge about X to identify a need for care, and must know that certain things could be done to improve the situation.

Condition II: S must choose and implement an action based on that knowledge, and intend the action to be a means for bringing about a positive change in X.

Condition III: The positive change must be judged solely on the basis of a "welfare-of-X" criterion.

To state these requirements in another way, any action may be described as caring if and only if S has identified a need for care and knows what to do for X, S chooses and implements an action intended to serve as a means for positive change in X, and the welfare-of-X criterion has been used to justify the choice and implementation of activities. There is a set of necessary relationships among the conditions. The intention or purpose of the chosen activity first must be related to the need for care and, second, must be intended to serve as a means of bringing about a positive change directly related to that need. The justification of the action as caring is then based on the nonarbitrary criterion: welfare-of-X.

This analysis provides a logical description of caring that included some action features. The next step in the analysis is to make even more explicit an action description of caring based on the conditions identified as being necessary for caring.

V. ACTION DESCRIPTION OF CARING

The theoretic description of caring as action was developed within the framework of the three previously identified conditions. The model used for the action description came from an action model of teaching developed by Kerr and Soltis.[19]

Caring as a Series of Actions

It would seem that caring, like teaching, is accomplished indirectly, that is, through many other activities, and in this sense may be considered mediated action. Consider, for example, the practice of nursing. While the goals of that health service are directed at caring activities that not only prevent, detect, and treat disease, but also promote and maintain health, no one activity of nursing (such as physical care, comfort measures, emotional support, or the like) could be considered the caring activity of nursing practice. What the following discussion explores is that caring, like teaching, is an intentional human enterprise, and as such is best discussed in terms of actions rather than specific caring behaviors.

Setting a Goal

One of the conditions essential to caring is related to the goal of bringing about a change in X in a positive direction. The condition reads: S must choose and implement an action intended to serve as a means for bringing about a positive change in X. If the goal of bringing about a positive change in X is necessary to speak of caring, then it would seem reasonable that any caring action would necessarily include the action of setting or recognizing a particular goal or goals relative to bringing about a positive change in X.

There are further considerations, however, in the action of setting a goal A(g) [Action (goal)], based on the condition that S not only must have enough knowledge about X to identify a need for care, but also must know what to do for X. If identification of a need for care is necessary to speak of S's caring for X, then any action called "caring" must also include some plan of activity or goal related to the identified need or needs.

Choosing A Tactic

At this point, S would be expected to choose the means or methods by which he or she intended to accomplish the particular goal. This action is one of choosing a tactic or tactics to achieve the goal—A(t) [Action (tactic)]. The term "tactic" is used to designate any method used to gain an end, especially short-range objectives. The tactic is chosen for the purpose of accomplishing the previously set goal and is implemented with that goal in mind.

Implementing The Tactic

What would count as an implementation of a tactic, A(i) [Action (implementation)], is determined by the tactic (t). Further consideration of the implementation activity [A (i)] requires that attention be given to the question of whether the activity implemented as a means or tactic (t) to achieve a goal (g) will in fact result in the accomplishment of that goal.

The likelihood that the chosen goal will be accomplished by the implementation of the chosen tactics, according to Kerr and Soltis, depends upon two factors:

> The likelihood that a particular activity will bring about achievement
> of some goal is at least based both on the chances in general that, *ceteris
> paribus*, the doing of the activity, will result in the achievement of the
> goal and on the person's mastery of that particular activity.[19]

While the mastery of an activity does not always result in the activity's being well executed, S's skill or mastery will undoubtedly affect the choice of appropriate tactics, which in turn affects the likelihood that the implementation of the activity will achieve the desired goal.

Thus far, the action description of S caring for X entails the actions of choosing a goal related to a need for care [A(g)], choosing tactics related to the achievement of the goal of bringing about a positive change in X [A(t)], and implementing the tactics [A(i)]. Certain factors are present in any caring situation that may impinge upon the actions described.

At least two further actions that provide a context for the mediated action series $A(g,t,i)$ must be considered. They are the action of setting a general goal $A(G)$, and the action of assessing the situation $A(S)$.

Setting a General Goal

The action of setting or recognizing a general goal concerns itself with the question: "On what basis might one decide what particular goals to achieve in relation to bringing about a positive change in X?" The action of setting a general goal, or recognizing a general goal previously set, according to Kerr and Soltis "provides or can provide a context for the mediated action series."[19] They further explained:

> Let us say that the action of setting or deciding upon a larger goal (G) is part of the context in which any teaching (or caring) takes place, but that it may be an empty action category, such as in the case in which the teacher decides on a whim rather than on a larger goal to pursue a particular learning goal (g).[19]

Assume that a nurse has identified a need for care and knows various ways to meet those needs. On what basis does she select a particular goal or goals to be accomplished? It would be reasonable to expect that the nurse would select particular goals that are part of a larger goal or goals directly related to the "welfare-of-X" criterion. For example, a general goal of nursing practice is to assist individuals and families to prevent or cope with the stress of illness and suffering. Within this goal (G), particular goals (g) are selected, and their accomplishment would assure the accomplishment of the general goal.

A recognized set of general goals (G) is not necessary, then, to every instance of caring as mediated action. Such general goals do, however, provide a context for the mediated action. One last action category to be considered also provides a context for the mediated action series—that of assessing the situation.

Assessing the Situation

Certain factors present in any caring situation may impinge upon the actions of choosing a goal, choosing a tactic, and implementing the tactic. Kerr and Soltis describe them as situational factors which need to be taken into account. The notation for the action of assessing situational factors reads: $A(S_1 \ldots S_n)$. For a better understanding of this action, let us consider the example of a nurse caring for a child with diabetes. The nurse sets the particular goal of getting the child to become more independent about his own care, and thus shorten the length of his stay in the hospital. She selects the activities that will serve as the tactic (t) by which to accomplish the goal (g). Activity A involves making the prospect of going to the playroom attractive to the child, and informing him that the option is open to him only under the condition that he test his own urine that morning (Activity B). From her experience and knowledge, the nurse knows that there is in general a good chance that this particular tactic will work. After having assessed the situation, however, she decides not to use that particular tactic. What factors might have led her to that decision? She may have learned that the child was to be discharged that afternoon; thus the goal of shortening the hospital stay no longer applied. Alternatively, she may have learned that the child is scheduled for surgery in the morning, thus changing the priority of the goal of "self-care." She may also have determined that the child had developed an infection, and visiting the playroom was no longer an option.

These considerations, and others like them, are situational factors that must be assessed prior to the choice and implementation of tactics. Assuming that the goals remain the same, the nurse must proceed to select another tactic with regard to the new situation.

If the particular goal must be changed, the nurse would initiate a new action series by setting a new goal.

Summary of Action Descriptions

Based upon the conditions necessary to speak of S's caring for X as a person, the following actions were identified to be necessary for a complete instance of S caring for X:

1. S chooses a particular goal or goals related to an identified need for care in X and the general goal (G) of positive change in X. This action is the first in a series of actions and is designated by the notation: $A(g_1 \ldots g_n)$.

2. S chooses tactics for the reason that they are likely to achieve the particular goal (g). Any activity may be considered a tactic if it is directly related to the accomplishment of the particular goal. This action is the second in the series and is designated by the notation: $A(t_1 \ldots t_n)$.

3. S implements the tactics by actually doing the activities chosen as tactics to accomplish the particular goal. This is the third and last in the series of caring actions and is designated by the notation: $A(i_1 \ldots i_n)$.

In notational form, this action description of caring reads: $[C: A(g_1 \ldots g_n),$ $A(t_1 \ldots t_n), A(i_1 \ldots i_n)]$. An essential connection occurs between the action constituents identified. For example, the choosing of a tactic is directly related to the particular goal (g $\longrightarrow$ t connection), and the implementation of a tactic is directly related to the tactic (t $\longrightarrow$ i connection). This connectedness permits us to discuss caring in an ordered series of actions beginning with goal-setting and ending with implementation.

The notation for this ordered series of actions in abbreviated form would read:

$$[C: A(g) \longrightarrow A(t) \longrightarrow A(i)]$$

A description of caring as an ordered series of actions is not complete without consideration of the action of setting a general goal [A(G)] and the action of assessing the situational factors [A(S)]. These two actions are directly connected to the action series [A(g, t, i)] in the sense that they impinge upon or provide a context for it. If there is any change in the perceived context that S considers relevant to the situation, then a new mediated action series would have to be initiated if the caring enterprise is to continue.

The action of choosing a particular goal [A(g)] within the context of overall goals [A(G)] establishes a $G \longrightarrow g$ connection. The goal selections [A(g) and A(G)] directly affect the choice and implementation of tactics—thus the [A(G) $\longrightarrow g \longrightarrow t \longrightarrow i$] connection. In much the same way, the action of choosing a tactic [A(t)] and the implementation of the tactic [A(i)] are directly influenced by the assessment of the situational factors [A(S)], thus establishing an [A(S) $\longrightarrow t \longrightarrow i$] connection. Of course, the situational factors also influence the feasibility of accomplishing the particular goal chosen, even to the point of requiring the setting of new goals. This then establishes an [A(S) $\longrightarrow g \longrightarrow t \longrightarrow i$)] connection.

The completed description of caring as an ordered series of actions [A(g), A(t), A(i)], within the context of the action categories of selection of general goals [A(G)] and assessing situational factors [A(S)], in full notation would read as follows:

$$C: A(G_1 \ldots G_n), A(S_1 \ldots S_n) / A(g_1 \ldots g_n),$$
$$A(t_1 \ldots t_n), A(i_1 \ldots i_n)$$

For convenience, or to emphasize the relationship among the action constituents, the following notation could be utilized:

Context

A(G)   A(S)

Caring: | A(g) $\longrightarrow$ A(t) $\longrightarrow$ A(i) |

Action Series

This theoretic description of caring, if it is an adequate description, should lead to the consideration of the question: "What must S do to be said to be skilled or competent in caring?"

V.   CARING COMPETENCY

Competency in General

The term "competency" is generally used to indicate the state or quality of having skill or abilities adequate for a specific purpose. The adverb "competently" applies only to those acts that a person intends to be a particular type of activity. For example, if Jane were to read a poem, it would not make sense to say that she was singing competently or incompetently, unless of course, she intended her actions to count as singing. Competence statements, then, can only be applied to purposive human action, as Kerr and Soltis noted when discussing teacher competency:

> Our concern with competence forces us to give serious and full attention to teaching as a purposeful human activity before judgments of competence or incompetence can be made . . . While it is possible to describe teaching, or any other human activity, as either action . . . or as behavior . . . our interest in competency advises an action description.[19]

If competency applies only to intentional activity, the question remains: "What particular activities must one be skilled in to be considered to be caring competently?" Caring is not a basic action that can be accomplished directly, but rather is a mediated action, accomplished through many other activities. Must one be skilled in all possible caring activities, or only particular ones? Exactly what skills might be considered caring competencies? To begin to answer, we will utilize the "caring as action" constituents identified previously in Section IV: The action of setting a goal or recognizing such a goal already set [A(g)], the action of choosing tactics to achieve the goal [A(t)], and the action of implementing the tactics [A(i)] within the context of setting a general goal [A(G)] and assessing the situation [A(S)].

Caring Competency

We begin with the last category in the action series, the action of implementing the tactic [A(i)]. The statement is made: "S (a nurse) performs that activity (communicating with X) very well." Would S be considered to be competently caring for X? To arrive at an answer to that question, it would be necessary to examine the related actions necessary for any caring action.

If caring can logically be considered an ordered series of actions, then to judge caring as being competent or incompetent based on only one activity—talking with S—would not seem reasonable. Although skill in the particular activities chosen to implement the tactic is required for competent action, there are other considerations to be made before stating that in a particular instance S was competently caring for X.

Competency in caring, then, can be assessed only if the particular action is intended to be a caring action, and such action includes:

1. The setting of particular goals that are related to overall goals (G $\longrightarrow$ g) intended to bring about a positive change in X.

2. The choosing of tactics for the purpose of accomplishing the goals (g ⟶ t). The "welfare-of-X" criterion would guide the choice of both goals and tactics.

3. Consideration of situational factors (identification of a specific need for care, to name one) prior to choosing and implementing tactics [A(S)/ (t ⟶ i)].

4. Implementation of the tactics with skill.

How competently one cares depends upon how well one does actions in the five categories: [A(G), A(S), A(g), A(t), A(i)], and how well one takes into account the other categories. The competencies for any instance of caring are to be found within the connections between the five action categories.

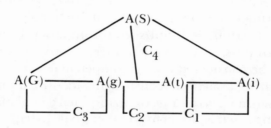

This notation enables one to grasp more fully the notion of the competencies existing within the action series.

The four competencies necessary for any instance of caring are as follows:

Competency I.   S implements the tactic well, or with skill [A(t) ⟶ A(i)].

Competency II.   S chooses a particular tactic for the right reasons; that is, the tactic is likely to accomplish the goal, and S is skilled in implementing the tactic [A(g) ⟶ A(t)].

Competency III.   S chooses goals that will lead to an overall goal; that is, the accomplishment of the particular goals will result in the accomplishment of an overall goal [A (G) ⟶ A(g)].

Competency IV.   S gives full consideration to the situational factors, that is, assesses the factors in the situation that may impinge upon the appropriateness of the goals, tactics, and implementation [A(S) ⟶ A(g ⟶ t ⟶ i)].

Given that S demonstrated, in any given instance of caring, the four competencies, the statement could be made that S was competent in caring for X.

However, what about the times S demonstrated only three of the four competencies required for caring, or perhaps did not demonstrate any competency in caring for Y and Z? It would seem that to consider S competent in caring, S must not only demonstrate some skill in the four competencies, but also be disposed to utilize those skills consistently over time with the persons he or she intends to care for in varying situations. That statement is not meant to imply, however, that if S demonstrated only three of the four competencies at any given time, S would be considered incompetent in caring.

Competent or incompetent caring, like caring or noncaring, is best thought of as a matter of degree, rather than as an absolute. Any instance of caring can be judged as competent or incompetent and may be attributed to certain skills, knowledges, and dispositions. The theoretic construct for caring as action offers a description of actions that may be judged as either caring or noncaring, competent or incompetent. The description goes beyond the identification of observable performative skills to include broader considerations of intention, choices, and judgments which underlie the performance.

Significance: The author offers the description of caring as a logical construct to which one can appeal for further discussions, especially of the determination and evaluation of caring in nursing.

Although the description does not offer a "how to teach caring" plan, it does serve as a framework for guiding the instructor in choosing goals and objectives related to caring action.

Future Plans for Research: The plan for future research is to develop a pilot empiric research project aimed at identifying, in naturalistic situations, "tactics" utilized by nurses who are recognized to be effective in various practice settings.

REFERENCES

1. Eriksen E: Identity, Youth and Crisis. New York, Norton, 1968 (1926).
2. Freud S: Inhibitions, Symptoms, Anxiety. London, Hogarth Press, 1966.
3. Fromm E: Man for Himself. New York, Rinehart, 1947.
4. Gaylin W: Caring. New York, Knopf, 1976.
5. Maslow A: Love in healthy people. *In* Montague A (ed.): The Practice of Love. Englewood Cliffs, NJ, Prentice-Hall, 1975, pp 89–113.
6. Eysenck HJ: The effects of psychotherapy. J Consult Psychol 16:319–324, 1952.
7. Levitt EE: The results of psychotherapy. J Consult Psychol 21:189–196, 1957.
8. Christensen CM: Relationships between pupil achievement, teacher warmth, and teacher-permissiveness. J Educ Psychol 51:169–174, 1959.
9. Pace CR, Stern GG: An approach to the measurement of physiological characteristics of college environment. J Educ Psychol 49:269–277, 1958.
10. Branstetter E: The young child's hospitalization. Communicating Nursing Research, WCHEN 2:1969.
11. Hadley BJ: Experimental trials of the nursing process. Communicating Nursing Research, WCHEN 17–39, 1975.
12. Johnson J, Dumas R, Johnson B: Interpersonal relations: the essence of nursing care. Nursing Forum 5(3):324–334, 1967.
13. Henry AM: Nurse behaviors perceived by patients as indicators of caring. Unpublished doctoral dissertation, Catholic University of America, 1975.

14. Leininger M: The phenomenon of caring: research questions and theoretical considerations. Paper presented at the First National Caring Conference, University of Utah, Salt Lake City, April 27 and 28, 1978. *In* Leininger M: Caring: An Essential Human Need. Thorofare, NJ, Slack Inc., 1981, pp 3–15.
15. Mayeroff M: On caring. Int Philos Q 5:462–474, 1965.
16. Nagel E: Philosophy in educational research. *In* Banghart FW: First Annual Symposium on Educational Research. Indiana, Phi Delta Kappa, 1960, p 75.
17. Peters RS: Ethics and Education. London, Allen and Unwin, 1966, p 16.
18. Scheffler I: Philosophy and Education. Boston, MA, Allyn and Bacon, 1958.
19. Kerr DH, Soltis JF: Locating teacher competency: an action description of teaching. Educational Therapy 24(1):3–16, Winter 1974.
20. Green TF: The Activities of Teaching. New York, McGraw-Hill, 1971.
21. Kaplan A: Conduct of Inquiry. Philadelphia, PA, Chandler Publishing Company, 1964, pp 332–358.

4

Caring: A Central Focus of Nursing and Health Care Services

INTRODUCTION

The case can be made that caring is the most important and central focus of nursing. Traditionally, nurses have used phrases such as, "I care," and "I gave nursing care to that patient." However, care has not been studied in a systematic way—a way that explores linguistic usage, epistemologic sources, and cross-cultural examples of care and their relationships to nursing. With this type of study, a scientific and humanistic body of nursing knowledge will result, which should improve client services by developing an in-depth perspective of the core of nursing.

Adopting a transcultural viewpoint, nurses can determine the nature, manifestations, and universal components of the diverse cultural groups in the United States and other lands. It is necessary to think of caring first in its anthropologic and historic dimensions and then to consider specific caring phenomena of the various cultures. As this large body of knowledge grows and comes together, nursing will have a solid, dynamic, and impressive base upon which to build education and practice. Most important, it will help validate and explain the distinct nature of nursing, which today tends to be vaguely understood, with many conflicting views about its essence. The knowledge will also be a contribution from nursing to other disciplines. It is hoped that a *science of caring* will develop and be used in helping people, social institutions, and cultures everywhere.

*Reprinted courtesy of Technomic Publishing Company, Westport, CT; October 1980 Nursing & Health Care, Madeleine M. Leininger, RN, PhD, FAAN, author. Man is used in a generic sense to refer also to women and children.

45

PART ONE

The author has hypothesized that throughout the remarkable history of Homo sapiens (more than one million years), caring for self and others has been the most critical factor that contributed to man's survival.[1] Caring for self and others in precarious and changing environments must have been a major daily human endeavor. Assisting individuals in need, helping the young and the weak, supporting the environmental risk-takers, and being aware of human growth and survival needs were important in early hominid lifeways. Today, these same caring needs are equally as important as we move into a new decade and soon into a new century.

The author's thesis is that caring is one of the most critical and essential ingredients for health, human development, human relatedness, well-being, and survival. She also contends that the concept that caring is essential to human survival and to human health and public services remains largely unknown and an area of systematic investigation that is neglected. It appears that caring as a human activity and capacity has been largely taken for granted until recently. It is indeed ironic that professional health disciplines speak about caring, but have not focused on the nature and essence of this phenomenon.

Definition, Nature, Usage and Importance of Human Caring

The term "care" as a noun generally refers to the attributes, actions, and qualities of assisting others in need. Webster's definition of care embodies the ideas of a felt interest in and concern for those who are in trouble, or wish to help those who are anxious, suffering, or facing uncertainties.[2]

For heuristic purposes, caring is defined in a generic sense as those human acts and processes that provide assistance to another individual or group based on an interest in or concern for that human being(s), or to meet an expressed, obvious, or anticipated need.[3] Professional caring embodies the cognitive and deliberate goals, processes, and acts of professional persons or groups providing assistance to others, and expressing attitudes and actions of concern for them, in order to support their well-being, alleviate undue discomforts, and meet obvious or anticipated needs. Professional nursing care is founded on this last definition but includes an emphasis on personalized caring from a holistic wellness and illness view of individuals, families, and community groups.

Another way to differentiate and understand caring is by referring to scientific and humanistic caring. Scientific caring refers to those judgments and acts of helping others based upon tested or verified knowledge; whereas humanistic caring refers to the creative, intuitive, or cognitive helping process for individuals or groups based upon philosophic, phenomenologic, and objective and subjective experiential feelings and acts of assisting others.[4]

In any caring process or context, it is important to consider the structural elements and functions of caregivers and care recipients, to understand their role and function, to realize what happens in caring situations, and to predict future caring encounters. The structural elements can be viewed as the predictive basis for continuity of care and for the way care becomes institutionalized as an ongoing human service. When individuals or groups seek health or human services, they generally find institutionalized values, actions, goals, and modes of caring. Such structural and functional elements constitute the cultural context of caring and are important areas of study in understanding the nature of institutional and professional services. The structure and organization of institutional care have been studied in a limited way.

Presently, there are diverse philosophic, linguistic, social, professional, and business ideas about care and caring as well as many ideas about what constitutes care. For example, it has been fascinating to note that in recent years business firms and other public service agencies have been using the term "care" in these phrases: "We care," "Caring is our business," "We care about you," "Caring's our service," and so on. It is evident that the professional usage of care has moved into the public domain, and this is encouraging banks, car dealers, and so forth, to care for people through their services. However, the forms, philosophy, and processes differ from nursing's professional services. With the public interest in care, we need a body of knowledge that can act as a stepping stone for more explicit and meaningful usage in the future.

The term "care" has been used by most health professional groups, and all have the freedom to use it. However, it has been the discipline of nursing that has used the term most persistently and continuously for more than a century. Since the beginning of modern nursing in the mid-1860s with Florence Nightingale's leadership and her book, *Notes on Nursing: What It Is and What It Is Not*, nurses have been charged to care for patients as whole persons.[5] Ms. Nightingale also emphasized health and the proper use of environmental resources. Christy, a nurse historian, states: "It is my opinion that Florence Nightingale saw the practice of nursing as far more important than the practice of medicine; when the physician cannot diagnose, he cannot care . . ."[6] The author has found that the physician often experiences considerable difficulty in being assistive to a patient's need for caring, especially with the incurably ill, for whom diagnosis or curative treatments are impossible. In contrast, professional nurses have never been limited in helping others through caring acts and processes, since they are not dependent upon medical diagnoses and treatments. The creative and skilled professional nurse can care for people without medical diagnoses and medical regimens. Moreover, the nurse can assist individuals, families, and cultural groups immediately with caring modalities and attitudes. The nurse can and does help individuals who are well, or who are under the threat of illness. This is the professional right and nature of the discipline of nursing, and one independent function that must be defended and not controlled or supervised by physicians. The public expects nurses to be caring (in the professional definition) and to assist people in need often beyond the physical level, such as the psychosocial and, more recently, the cultural areas.

While the term "nursing care" has been used many years, it is evident that the concept of care, with its divergent linguistic usages, has not been systematically studied by nurses in a rigorous and persistent manner. In another publication, the author stated;

> One of the most essential, promising, and important areas of study in nursing is the concept of caring, and yet, it has been one of the most neglected areas of systematic research. Although nurses are the professional group who repeatedly use the expressions "nursing care," "care" and "caring" in everyday parlance, the linguistic, semantic, and professional usages of these terms are still limitedly understood and studied.[7]

It is paradoxic that nurses have not investigated a term that they use daily and by which they would be expected to defend their professional activities. Nursing faculty, students, and clinical staff can offer many meanings of care, most of which are their personal views rather than concepts or theories that have undergone rigorous investigation. Likewise, "medical care" and "dental care" have diverse usages and meanings which may bear study by those disciplines.

The author began to study the phenomenon of care in the late 1950s. However, she soon discovered that there were cultural differences in the perceptions of care, which led her to study cultural anthropology in 1959.

Cross-Cultural Interests, Questions, and Research Findings

The author's study of anthropology led to questions about the role of caring and curing in human evolution and survival of the human species. Observation of medical practice revealed a discipline that has been oriented toward curing with focus on physical diagnoses, internal pathology and treatments aimed at cure. In contrast, nursing was directed at caring acts and processes focusing on multiple factors influencing wellness and illness. While nursing was aware of some internal body conditions, more interest was properly placed on external factors that maintain wellness and prevent illnesses.[8] This conceptual and professional difference between the disciplines needed to be examined from an anthropologic view to identify patterns of human caring and curing. Furthermore, the author hypothesized that caring acts and processes must have been critical to early man's development and survival. Curing played a role but was not as essential as caring.

Virtually nothing explicit on caring behaviors and no theories in the anthropology literature on caring were found. There were some descriptive statements that could be interpreted as caring, but no substantive knowledge or firm documentation. There were, however, ethnographic descriptions of curing, most of these made by male curers. The absence of caring indicators led the author to develop philosophic and epistemologic ideas about caring.

To begin, it was theorized that caring must have been imperative for prehistoric man to survive in rugged and precarious environments. Presumably, mother or mother surrogate played a key role in nurturing, protecting, defending, and instructing her offspring. What role did males play in caring, however, since early man lived in hordes, nomadic bands, or loose social and familylike groups? What role did caring acts play in developing and reinforcing social ties, social organization, and cultural norms? Was caring the mode used to protect groups from external human and environmental threats? It was postulated that sharing of food, material goods, tools, and even men, women, and children were acts of caring for others who had limited resources and needed physical and human help. Were these caring acts? If so, were they a prototype of altruism which led to present-day social and cultural exchanges and gift-giving? Practically speaking, what happened when men, women, and children became ill, injured, or disabled? Who cared for them when they were ill? Most important, do the caring elements we find in modern nursing exist by virtue of human nature and culturally constituted behavior? Unfortunately, these theoretic statements and questions are unanswered. They have kept nurse-anthropologists busy exploring ideas related to each question about early forms of human caring.

In 1965, the author discovered that nurses' ideas of caring and those of patients differ. An ongoing study of 30 cultures regarding nurses' perceptions and knowledge about caring behaviors, processes, roles, and techniques and those of care recipients evolved to establish ethnonursing data about caregivers and receivers.[9] Using the ethnoscience approach with linguistic, ethnographic, and clinical data, some preliminary findings can be shared.

First: Professional caring behaviors, activities, and processes varied considerably among nurses of different cultural backgrounds. Their caring perceptions and activities regarding clients of the same and different cultures deviated.[24] Nurses in different cultures tend to know and emphasize different care constructs such as support, comfort, and touch. For example, in the United States, Anglo-American nurses perceive that one of their dominant duties is to alleviate stress through technologic aids, medicines, and psychophysiologic comfort measures. In several non-Western cultures, nurses and clients perceive care as protective and surveillance acts and processes, largely with a sociocultural emphasis. For example, Samoan caregivers are expected to protect clients from breaking cultural and social rules in order to prevent illness or harm to clients. Preliminary findings also show more congruence between the expectations of care recipients and caregivers in non-Western than in Western societies. For example, in the United States there appears to be a wide cultural gap between nurses' perceptions of what constitute caring acts and those of the public. This is a wider cultural gap than in Western Samoa.

Second: The concept of helping or assisting others in need, or anticipating the needs of care recipients, was evident among all caregiving nurses, and most care recipients expected nurses to help them or anticipate their needs. To date, we have found no universal cross-cultural definition of professional caring, but there are common descriptive terms that support definitions already cited. There are, however, many different ideas about components of care in the 30 cultures, such as the following: comfort, support, attention, compassion, touch, love, protection, surveillance, personalized help, nurture, stress alleviation, restoration, tenderness, trust, instruction, maintaining well-being, succor, empathy, direct assistance (or helping acts), stimulation, helping the dependent, presence, and medical-technical assistance.[9]

Each of these ideas about caring varied in emphasis, and some were not used or known in certain cultures. In most of the cultures, professional nurses were able to give priority to the caring ideas they valued most as caregivers. For example, Anglo-American nurses emphasized stress alleviation using psychophysiologic acts and processes, whereas Chinese nurses saw surveillance and protection as the dominant caring mode. In some cultures, touch was to be avoided except in emergency or special circumstances. In New Guinea, the professional caregivers considered prevention, surveillance, and instruction to be of equal and related importance; these caregivers emphasize prevention and health maintenance. This follows the tradition of folk caregivers' helping people long before the professional caregivers (nurses) came into existence. This was especially true with vulnerable infants and adults in the culture.[10]

Third: Ethnoscientific and ethnographic data revealed that caring behaviors were mainly provided by female caregivers (both professionals and nonprofessionals), and males were associated with cure-giving behaviors. In non-Western and Western societies, most male cure-givers were in the field of medicine. This finding supports the theory that medicine emphasizes curing acts, while nursing tends to emphasize caring activities. In the 30 cultures studied, the folk health-illness systems tended to dichotomize caring and curing roles, and they linked males with the curing role and females with more caring responsibilities. There were, however, signs of change occurring, with more women entering medicine and men nursing, especially in Western cultures such as the United States. In Russia and China, there is a large number of women in medicine, environmental health, and prevention.

Fourth: Caring behaviors and processes appear closely related to, and could be understood by, social structure in most cultures. For example, nurses from Israel and Turkey related their caring functions to restorative activities due to frequent war and changing economic factors. The New Guinean, Samoan, and Fijian care activities of protection and surveillance appeared closely linked to their religious and kinship structure as well as to cultural beliefs about sorcery and ancestral spirits. Likewise, the indigenous caregivers held similar roles in the past—to prevent illness and to maintain health by reinforcing cultural taboos and practices of daily life. In contrast, Anglo-American nurses in the United States were closely linked to educational, medical, and technologic features of social structure. The interrelationship between social structure and nursing care practices is a largely new and fascinating area for future investigation, which would well provide predictive and prescriptive bases for nursing care practices.

Fifth: Ritualistic caring acts exist in all cultures in their symbolic and nonsymbolic methods of helping people. In several non-Western cultures, the professional rituals were congruent with the folk practices, whereas in Western society there were signs of incongruencies. In some Western cultures, the caregivers were active participants in the caring rituals. Mexican-American folk caregivers employed the mal ojo (the evil eye) ritual to restore the sick child; professional Mexican-American nurses understood this ritual, but did not practice it in hospitals (although some did in the home). Many caring rituals of a technologic and psychophysiologic nature could be identified in Western societies such as the United States by their desired therapeutic outcomes. For example, rituals in feeding children, in cardiovascular resuscitation, and in mental health therapies were mentioned for therapeutic purposes.

The cross-cultural study of therapeutic and nontherapeutic caring rituals is another rich area, especially in linking folk and professional health services together in a meaningful way. During the past several years, graduate seminars on folk and professional caring rituals have been conducted. Participating students soon realized that there are a growing number and variety of ritualistic activities in our American hospitals—actually increasing each year. The therapeutic functions of ritualistic activities in caring should be studied frequently for their merits and for health maintenance and prevention. Throughout time, rituals have been important in health care. In the future we need to emphasize certain ones, such as exercise rituals, and change others, such as eating rituals for obese persons. In our American hospitals, the childbirth ritual of positioning the mother in labor on her back contrasts sharply with many cultures in the world in which mothers are positioned kneeling or squatting, rather than lying on a hospital delivery table. The consequence of this unnatural position for the client must be questioned; it was instituted in England to serve the obstetrician rather than the comfort of the patient. This position may lead to postdelivery back pains and leg discomfort due to the very awkward positioning of the client, which does not support the body structure of humans from a physical anthropologic stance.

Several other rituals also need to be reviewed for their therapeutic value and to determine whom they serve the most. In addition, hospital and other human services need to examine their helpful and less helpful rituals.

Sixth: From the ethnographic and research findings from the 30 cultures, it has been theorized that due to the advent of modern scientific medicine and medical practices, the local or nonmedical consumers are finding professional knowledge and practices to be too complex, too questionable, and too geographically inaccessible, especially for poor and middle to lower socioeconomic groups. Hence, a cultural gap has occurred, with folk practices increasing. We are aware that the cost of scientific medicine has increased, so that many poor people are unable to purchase the services, treatments, and medications. Most important, some physician treatments and regimens do not make sense to certain cultural groups, especially related to their views of the cause and way to treat a health problem. Frequently, physicians and other professional health personnel do not know folk illnesses and their treatment. Some dismiss them in a demeaning way, and this causes problems of distrust.

Those cultures that are reactivating or continuing to use their folk health system contend that their treatment ways are: easily accessible (generally located in their home community), readily understood in their cultural life context; and truly holistic (treating the whole person rather than organs). Local folk practitioners can participate directly in all care and treatment, and folk care services can be obtained at much lower costs than professional medical services.[11] In general, professional health services tend to be sought last by cultural minority groups after local or folk health services fail. Hence, there is a growing gap between professional health systems and folk health practices, and there is a lack of knowledge on the part of professional staff regarding how folk practices serve clients. There is a need to link folk and professional caregiving and receiving practices.

With the new subfield of transcultural nursing, nurses who have gained a knowledge of the differences between folk and professional care can help make meaningful links with clients. In fact, some nursing students are taking active steps to incorporate the indigenous folk healers into professional health care. For example, in one of the Navaho nursing care services, the medicine man or singers are active participants in hospital care services, and Navajo mothers are encouraged to use their infant cradle boards and to be at home for their blessing ceremonies. As a consequence, professional nurses are learning the values and functions of folk health maintenance and prevention, and particularly how folk practices can complement professional caring and curing to provide better health care. Transcultural awareness helps nurses use anthropologic and nursing knowledge creatively to work with people of different cultural backgrounds and to provide culture-specific nursing care. A similar culturologic approach is needed in medicine, dentistry, and other health disciplines to provide meaningful care.

PART TWO

Epistemologic, Philosophic, and Theoretic Considerations

In this next section, some general epistemologic, philosophic, and theoretic statements are made to stimulate thinking along future lines of investigation related to caring. From inferential interdisciplinary sources, one can theorize that caring activities and processes were essential in the past for human survival, development, growth, wellness, recovery, and social relatedness. They remain so today. Biocultural data on the evolution of mammals supports the idea that the young are helpless and dependent creatures who need the support of adults for protection and survival. This epistemologic premise gains support from psychologic anthropology and from the psychologic view that it is important to socialize the young in a conscientious way so that they will survive, learn desired cultural values, and transmit the norms to succeeding generations. Concepts related to maintaining wellness and preventing illness with specific techniques of caring must have existed in the past; they form the epistemologic and philosophic base for a science of caring in nursing and the health fields. This assumption is only inferred and needs further documentation.

In recent years, the author has encouraged nurses to focus on caring and to develop both humanistic and scientific bases for nursing care. The work of Watson, Ray, Travelbee, Bevis, and Leininger, along with National Caring Conferences held since 1978, have helped explain caring behaviors and processes and new lines of research.[8,12-16] The cross-cultural focus is providing valuable data on which to base nursing care theories.

In searching further for knowledge sources regarding human caring, ideas from psychology, religion, nursing, biology, ecology, and other sources have been noted. A combined psychoanalytic, biologic, and culturologic explanation is offered by Gaylin about caring in response to the infant's dependent, powerless, and helpless nature:

> To be helpless and unloved is the matrix of disaster. The "poser" of helplessness fuses with the "power" of loving ability to become an essential part of the complicated dependency lessons that the infant will almost inevitably carry into his adult life.[17]

Nurses frequently observe the parents' capacity to care for and love their offspring. Nurses have also visited in homes where parents physically and psychologically abuse, harm, or kill their children. The author believes that the insecurity of parents and the lack of preparation for parenthood play a major role in child abuse. Caring must be learned, and parents need to develop an interest in and capacity for caring. Still another theory is that the infant learns about caring and his culture immediately after birth; learning and caring experiences begin in the hospital with the nurse. The nurse's touching, holding, protecting, and feeding are some of the early caring activities. Because the nurse and the mother (and sometimes the father) are the main caregivers, we should investigate the caring modes of nurses that facilitate a positive caring environment. The hospital as a caring environment is another important focus for study.

It is important to review the works of philosophers, psychologists, and other health professionals related to caring. *The Art of Loving, Love and Will,* and *Caring* contribute insights about caring expressed through the concepts of love, self-growth, identification, hope, development of a human conscience, attachment, self-awareness, and other human expressions.[11,18,19]

Mayeroff's philosophic treatise sees caring as more than an interest in another human. He speaks about caring as an important means for self-growth through helping others:

> To help another person grow is at least to help him to care for something or someone apart from himself, and it involves encouraging and assisting him to find and create of his own in which he is able to care. Also, it is to help that other person to come to care for himself, and by becoming responsive to his own needs to care and to become responsible for his own life.[20]

Caring can be inferred from the works of phenomenologists, existentialists, and philosophers by an analysis of their perceptions and cognitions. Their writings about presence, being, experiencing, loving, perceptual sets, and intuitive feelings can be used to develop, test, and understand concepts of caring in health and human services.[21],[22]

Religious philosophers and theologians also consider aspects of caring as a religious obligation and expect that people will gather as God's own in a loving and concerned way to fulfill His will. In religious teachings and in the Bible, caring and loving are linked together with the expectation that people will love and care for one another as God's children. People are expected to help others, sacrifice for one another, and watch over and protect each other with a caring attitude. Writings of humanists, poets, artists, and social scientists often provide many descriptors that infer caring, such as: compassion, sympathy, empathy, love, expressive lifestyles, "humanness," relatedness, helpfulness, and shared mutual life experiences. Thus, there are many ideas related to the generic definition of caring that appear to be essential and desirable for human growing and living together to fulfill aspirations, goals, and dreams. These seminal ideas can be used to develop caring further in human services.

Curing is Additive to Caring

Turning to some specific theories about caring, the author contends that there can be no curing without caring, but there may be caring without curing.[7] This theoretic position is based upon repeated observations by the author as a professional nurse and upon logical inferences. She finds that caring is essential to curing and pervades all efforts to help an individual recover after an illness. Most important, caring can occur without curing; this can be observed repeatedly in clinical nursing practice. From cross-cultural data, we learned that patients in the Republic of China must be prepared mentally by means of a caring attitude before and after curing treatments occur. These caring attitudes are accomplished by involving the patient in social activities, eating with the patient, and supporting him. In many cultures, nurses care for patients without curing intent and with no medical curing treatments or regimens. In America, the author contends that for years professional nurses have provided many caring acts and decisions for clients in the home, school, industries, and hospitals. Medical curing acts are additive to the caring process. Sometimes caring and curing may support and reinforce each other and thus are difficult to separate. However, we need to separate caring activities and their therapeutic effects from curing to know and understand them better.

According to Becker et al, it appears that only a small number of people who come for services are cured.[23] The more one thinks about and observes people with health problems, the more one realizes that caring should be the major emphasis of all health and nursing care services. Nurses, as the largest group of health care providers, could and should make a major difference in health services if caring were the focus of their practice. The author contends that since most clients come to hospitals in the United States (expect for short-term emergencies) to receive caring, we need to give far more attention to this process than presently occurs. This position seems understandable, for often clients have been to physician's offices for cures prior to being hospitalized. Generally, these clients know their diagnosis and prognosis and have received medical treatments before entering the hospital. Upon admission, they want to receive good care, such as rest, being listened to, being observed, and being helped in many other ways by competent nurses. Thus, the hospital should emphasize caring as a dominant service. Presently, the opposite seems evident, with far more focus on curing aspects in medical treatment regimens. As we give more emphasis to caring, we will discover how clients remain well and prevent illnesses. The nursing profession must lead this shift of emphasis and must value caring as an important human health service.

Presently, there is virtually no price placed on caring in our society. Costs are primarily focused on medical curing and physician services related to medical diagnoses, treatments, and medications. Although very little economic value is assigned to caring, the author estimates that three-fourths of health services are caring and only one-fourth curing. Logically, more recognition and economic worth must be placed on caring, especially on caring as a preventive and health maintenance mode, along with sharper delineation in all sectors of health education.

Caring as a Central Thrust of Research

This leads to the author's philosophy that caring behaviors, processes, and structures are the central and most unifying focus of nursing practice, and should comprise the major intellectual, theoretic, practical, and research endeavors of nurses.[9] While the nursing profession has expressed interest in caring for people from a holistic health view, nurses have not pursued the phenomenon of care with any intellectual and practical rigor. Many have been too involved in medical magic and curing methods. It is time to focus on caring for people. While other diverse ideas about nursing exist, such as time, self-care, system behavior, and so forth, the author maintains that nursing's most singular and unique contribution to society is caring for human beings. This concept makes sense out of all nursing activities.

There is a need for support by nursing leadership, both in education and practice, to focus on caring and to get about the business of caring. In the past decade, nursing students have been eager to become more active in and excited about studying specific caring constructs such as support, comfort, and touch, as well as studying hospitals as caring institutions. They need, however, faculty and nursing leaders who are committed to caring rather than medical activities. Again, in the past few years nursing curricula have just been beginning to focus on caring as the central curriculum, theory, and research focus. There is a gradual shift from studying medical disease entities, diagnoses, and pathologies to studying nursing care entities, assessments, and processes. Whether caring constructs and practices will become a part of teaching, practice, and research depends largely upon the commitment of nursing to study and demonstrate caring behaviors. Indeed, the author also contends that the real research of nursing will focus on caring and nursing care rather than on physiologic, sociologic, psychologic, and anthropologic domains of knowledge per se. Today there are far too many research studies that are extremely remote from nursing and caring practices. The author believes that these studies exist because nurses do not understand and value caring.

Quantifying Effectiveness

Closely related to understanding caring is the author's theoretic position that recovery from illnesses, acceptance of death, and maintenance of human well-being are largely contingent upon cognitive nursing care processes and goals. While many nurses may hold this statement to be true, research is far too scanty to validate the theory. Studies demonstrating the difference that professional nursing care makes on individual and family recovery and well-being are urgently needed. New ways of helping also need to be recognized. Nurses may be the innovators of new health practices, but their ideas are quickly taken over by others, providing limited opportunity to study what difference nursing care ideas can make in the helping process. For example, we are aware that the hospice movement in England began with a professional nurse who wished to help clients and their families accept incurable types of body illnesses and to help them during the dying process. In the United States, several of our hospices were started and established by professional nurses to provide health and nursing care services for clients with incurable illnesses. All too frequently, these kinds of care centers (and others), which are launched to provide better services to individuals and families, are taken over by business groups, industrial enterprises, or physicians; financial pressures are often the reason. Consequently, these noteworthy projects can change from caring to noncaring financial enterprises under medical control. This is comparable to what has happened with some nursing care homes and other innovative services launched by nurses. We face problems in trying to maintain and control health and nursing care services that are nurse-operated. The few centers that have survived, such as our University of Utah nursing-centered clinics (including the large Navajo Project) and the Loeb Center, have required very strong leadership and resources in an environment of economic and political control. Economic and public support for such innovative, cost-effective, and therapeutic care is needed to demonstrate how nursing care influences recovery, health maintenance, and the well-being of individuals and families.

Nonsexist Caregiving

Another theoretic position is that caring can be provided in different ways by both female and male caregivers through learned socialization processes. Ethnographic and ethnonursing literature from the past describes females as the primary caregivers and males as curers. While this pattern has existed in the past, the author finds insufficient indicators and arguments to support caregiving as being limited to and given more effectively by females. While female caring and male curing activities in nursing and the 30 cultures studied have been described, these appear to be linked with past cultural norms and practices.[9,24] Traditionally, caregiving has been linked primarily to women in the home who are feeding, nurturing, caressing, and providing direct care to offspring, whereas males performed nonhouse and nonchildcaring activities. Social status and division of labor along sex roles were evident. Male caregivers in the nursing profession are equallly as competent in their roles and can learn and use caring constructs. Male caregivers must, however, have opportunities to learn role attributes such as nurturing, caressing, comforting, and compassion. In our schools of nursing, we are finding some "mid-husbands" surpassing midwives in expressive caring behaviors. The cross-cultural arguments (based on biologic and genetic factors) that only females can be caring by virtue of the fact that they bear children and assume domestic roles have limited support today. In general, the author believes that caring is essentially a culturally learned and expressed behavior.

The Future

Because people desire human caring or its comparable attributes, caring will receive more emphasis in the human services despite countercultural forces. Individuals who learn to value caring as strength will negotiate for humanistic care services and settings, for lacking care, human beings will behave in more animal-like ways, and an atmosphere of apathy, hostility, despair, and war can prevail.

To teach caring is to learn what it is. To learn about caring requires researching its roots and tracing their progeny. Our challenge is the development of caring people, caring cultures, and caring social institutions. Why not make caring work effectively in the United States so that we could serve as an example to other cultures that may be having difficulty in valuing and understanding human rights, human justice, and human caring?

The Challenge

Systematic research to describe caring behavior, values, and practices in nursing and other health professions clearly is needed so that incorporation of that knowledge into education and practice systems can take place.

Meanwhile, counterproductive forces continue to hinder humanistic values.

Technology threatens human concerns. Marc Lelonde, a Canadian health leader, states that health professionals regard the human body as a machine which is kept running by replacing or removing defective parts or clearing clogged lines.[25] Furthermore, health care settings strive for efficiency, standardization, and routine, which undermines the very nature of the client system to be served, and which risks treating people like robots.

Economic worth has not been traditionally associated with caring; there is no item in the budget for "care." Possibly, the role of women as the major caregivers who have provided care without cost has limited economic reward in the health occupations. We wonder how much professional caring is worth, how care is valued vis-à-vis curing, and how the economic value of female caregivers in our country and elsewhere can be changed.

Dehumanizing bureaucratic practices of our social institutions—hospitals, schools, and public agencies—need transformation. Nursing can act as the change agent to establish the institution and all levels of staff as sources of caring. Nurses will need to work with research findings to educate administrators, staff, and students in the humanizing of their health care settings. The end product should be a public view of the institution as humanistic, based on a reality brought about by nurses as caring professionals.

For survival, human development, self-actualization, and human relatedness to occur, care needs to occur. Definition of attributes, recognition of the caregiver's worth, and integration of an operational philosophy of caring in health institutions have only begun. It is a humanistic philosophy that permits exploration of caring and development of the *science of caring*. This will help us understand more fully how caring in human services binds us together in this society and how human beings are linked together as one great culture.

REFERENCES

1. Leininger M: The phenomenon of caring: the essence and central focus of nursing. American Nurses' Foundation (Nursing Research Report) 12(1):1977, pp 2,14.
2. Merriam W: Webster's New Collegiate Dictionary. Springfield, MA, G.P. Merriam Co., 1975, p 168.
3. Leininger M: Cross-cultural functions of caring and nursing care In Leininger M(ed): Proceedings of the Second National Caring Conference. Salt Lake City, UT, 1980.
4. Leininger M: Humanism, health and cultural values. Health Care Dimensions. Philadelphia, PA, F.A. Davis Co., 1974, pp 37–60.
5. Nightingale F: Notes on Nursing: What It Is and What It Is Not. New York, D. Appleton and Company, 1860, pp 1–2.
6. Christy T: Nursing: historical perspectives of a proud profession or how we got here from there. Unpublished paper of Keynote Address to the Pennsylvania Nurses' Association, Pennsylvania, October 4, 1976, p 3.
7. Leininger M: Some philosophical, historical and contemporary perspectives about caring phenomena in the American nursing culture. Paper presented at the Third National Caring Conference, Salt Lake City, UT, March 18, 1980.
8. Leininger M: Cross-cultural ethnonursing study of caring behaviors, processes and linguistic usages in western and non-western societies. Unpublished ongoing research. Salt Lake City, UT and Seattle, WA, 1965–1980.
9. Leininger M: Transcultural Nursing: Concepts, Theories, and Practices. New York, Wiley & Sons, 1978, pp 39–45.
10. Leininger M: The Gadsup of New Guinea and the early child-caring behaviors with nursing care implications. Transcultural Nursing Care of Infants and Children. Proceedings of the First National Transcultural Nursing Conference, Salt Lake City, UT, 1976, pp 201–219.
11. Leininger M: Consumer health care needs, nursing leadership and future directions. Proceedings of the Leadership in Nursing Conference. Seattle, University of Washington School of Nursing, 1979.

12. Watson J: Nursing: The Philosophy and Science of Caring. Boston, MA, Little, Brown & Co., 1979.
13. Ray MA: A philosophical analysis of caring. Unpublished paper for Second National Caring Conference, Salt Lake City, UT, 1978.
14. Travelbee J: Interpersonal Aspects of Nursing. Philadelphia, PA, F.A. Davis Co., 1971
15. Bevis EO: Conceptual framework: the knowledge component. Curriculum Building in Nursing: A Process. 2nd ed. St. Louis, MO, C.V. Mosby Co., 1978, pp 110–122.
16. Leininger M: Chairperson, National Caring Conferences, Salt Lake City, UT, 1978, 1979, 1980.
17. Gaylin W: Caring. New York, Avon Books, 1976, p 44.
18. Fromm E: The Art of Loving, New York, Bantam Books, 1956, p 33.
19. May R: Love and Will. New York, Morton, 1969.
20. Mayeroff M: On Caring. New York, Harper & Row, 1971.
21. Marcel G: Presence and Immortality. Pittsburgh, PA, Duquesne University Press, 1967.
22. Teilhard D: On Love, New York, Harper & Row, 1967.
23. Becker M(ed): The health belief model and personal health behavior. Health Education Monograph 2:4, 1974.
24. Leininger M: Transcultural caring and nursing care behaviors with taxonomy of 30 cultures. Unpublished ongoing research. Salt Lake City, UT and Seattle, WA, 1974 to present.
25. Lalonde M: A New Perspective on the Health of Canadians. A Working Document, Ottawa, Ontario, Government of Canada, 1974.

5

Motivational and Historical Aspects of Care and Nursing

The term "nursing care" has been used traditionally to denote a service rendered by nurses to those with illness-related needs. However, there has been a lack of clarity regarding the necessary characteristics of such service. Viewpoints range from the position that nursing care is identified by specific prescribed procedures performed by one who is designated as nurse, to the broader perspective that nursing care encompasses a fuller scope of interaction and involvement between nurse and patient.[1]

In this chapter, a distinction is made between the polarities of understanding regarding nursing care. The term *nursing care* refers to the performance of specific procedures by nurses; whereas the phrase *caring in nursing* denotes the totality of service rendered through nurse-patient interactions.

Societal recognition and compensation of nursing services have traditionally been for nursing task performance rather than comprehensive nursing intervention. However, there has been a commonly held expectation that personal traits and attitudes conveyed by the nurse should in fact contribute to the care-receiver's experienced sense of satisfaction. Such anticipation of subjectively satisfying caring experiences has often been frustrated for both caregivers and care-receivers, as external regulations and controls have served to govern nursing practice settings.

As a consequence, some nurses are increasingly seeking to justify such concomitant caring expression in task performance as a legitimate part of nursing practice. However, ambiguity exists in our understanding of the concept of caring, because it has developed for the most part in response to societal norms, religious beliefs and values, and economic and political policies rather than from direct study of the underlying principles involved in the nurturing aspects of life.[1-3]

Nursing's recent focus on the concept of caring has been encouraged by growing societal concern about the increased technologic emphases of health care and other directions of the behavioral sciences.

It is appropriate and timely that such heretofore silent areas of knowledge about caring be recognized, formalized, and explicated.[1,2] Past ideas of caring have largely been shaped and directed by philosophic systems that have, in turn, been influenced by the provincialisms of particular times and places in history. It may be that past perceptions of caring may not be entirely appropriate and useful for society at this present time.

A survey of the literature indicates that in the past, caring has been advocated and encouraged through moral directives to caregivers. The prevalence of such directives has implied that caring attitudes and behaviors are inherent in effective nursing practice. However, utilizing a moral approach to caring has resulted in an avoidance of dealing with the question of how to actualize caring attitudes and behaviors consistently in nursing practice.

One problem with associating the concept of caring with moralistic dimensions has been raised by Dickoff and James, who pointed out that problems can arise when thought is not linked to action, or when action is not guided by thought.

> The two modes of philosophic sin are particularly related to beliefs and values, for all too often values or ideas are merely heady abstractions unrealized and unrealizable in action; and, moreover, many of the principles that guide action are beliefs more like dogmas or catechism responses than like verbalizations produced as a product of, or guide to, action.[4]

Dickoff and James further noted that despair results when ideals are not realized either because external circumstances make them unrealizable or because the agents lack the energy or capacity for their realization. Scrutinizing ideals in search of discrepancies between thought, verbalization, and action can serve as a therapy for the despair caused by unsatisfied or unrealized ideals.

A second problem with viewing caring solely from moralistic perspectives is that it ignores the possibility that caring may be viewed as an empiric inquiry that is amenable to scientific study, or as a formal philosophic question. Without a systematic approach to the study of caring, it is possible for ambiguous subjective speculations to be used inaccurately as philosophic reasonings or as pseudoscientific theorizing.

Another problem that may arise in the absence of updated knowledge about caring is the potential for trivializing a significant aspect of human interaction as the concept of caring is adopted for the promotion of marketable goods and services (eg, "Credit Unions CARE about you" and "WDGY—the station that CARES"). Titmuss has pointed out that there is potential for distortion and exploitation when a human transaction that has traditionally been a gift relationship comes to be viewed as a marketable commodity within a competitive economic system.[5] The occurrence of such an untoward effect is more likely to be seen when there is inadequate knowledge available for appropriate use in unfamiliar situations, according to Titmuss.

Because understanding interpersonal relationships has been seen as significant to understanding caring, there has been a tendency to look primarily to the fields of psychology and sociology as resources for studying caring. However, it is appropriate that the discipline of nursing, which has traditionally been associated with caring roles and behaviors, should explore the concept of caring from within its own historic framework. Identifying and analyzing past perceptions and insights about caring in nursing can provide a baseline for empiric inquiry that is amenable to further research into the concept of caring.

MOTIVATION AS A COMPONENT OF CARING

Caring in nursing has been conceptualized in the literature in terms of moral, cognitive, and innate aspects of motivation.

The descriptive phrase, "moral/cognitive/innate motivation" is used in this study to denote the beliefs and values that have encouraged individuals or groups to participate in caring behaviors in nursing.

In this description, "moral" denotes conforming to a standard of right behavior that is sanctioned by or operative on one's conscience or ethical judgment.

"Cognition" is defined as (1) knowledge based on or capable of being reduced to empiric facts or (2) the act or process of knowing, including both awareness and judgment.

"Innate" refers to the inherent or essential genetically determined nature of an individual.

"Motivation" indicates a stimulus to action or an inducement that causes a person or group to act.

Differentiation between moral, cognitive, and innate perspectives of motivation for caring in nursing are not stated directly in the literature, but are instead found through examination of contextual material. For the most part, references to motivation for caring are made through such terms as duty, service, obligation, devotion, commitment, benevolence, compassion, charity, and pity. Such references indicate that there is consensus regarding the significance of being concerned about the distress of others and being willing to alleviate such distress. In fact, on first reading it may appear that motivation for caring is indeed composed of this sense of concern for others. However, further reading reveals that there are underlying factors which can be seen as providing the stimulus for such concern about the well-being of others. Examples are presented here to illustrate three aspects of motivation that are depicted in the literature.

Moral Aspects of Motivation

Moral aspects of motivation for caring in nursing are usually emphasized in nursing histories whose authors have observed rather than participated in nursing. For example, Saunders alluded to moral motivation as he sought to describe the fundamental core of nursing from the perspective of sociology:

> Whenever and wherever the nursing function is performed, there are always present two indispensable components, the patient and the nurse—one needing, one giving. The continuity, the stability, the enduring quality of nursing is to be found here in the never-failing willingness of some people to give that others may have—to provide for those who need the relief from pain, comfort, assurance, support, and, perhaps more important than any of these, the sense that there is someone who knows, someone who understands, someone who cares.[6]

Saunders' intention was to identify objectively the fundamental core of nursing through the scientific perspective of sociology. However, he instead assumed the popularized societal position that the norm for motivation for caring is comparable with the commitment that is usually associated with religious vows and ideal views on moral discipline.

Moral and Cognitive Aspects of Motivation

Nurse-authors have also alluded to moral aspects of motivation, but usually in combination with inferences to cognitive aspects. Nutting and Dock traced the historic growth of nursing toward a scientific discipline, and thus pointed out cognitive aspects of motivation that were based on empiric nursing knowledge and the desire to achieve a nonmoral good or goal.[7] Although they attempted to differentiate scientific nursing values from traditional moral beliefs of their time, they in effect linked the two aspects of motivation.

As historians, Nutting and Dock emphasized that Nightingale's work during the Crimean War was not limited to a popularized notion of "the lady with the lamp":

> Gone forever, from the time when she applied her intellect to the problems of the Crimea, was the conception of nursing as a charity, exceedingly meritorious and deserving of the heavenly reward for its self-sacrificing character. The self-sacrifice remained, but under her sway nursing shone forth as a part of the science of health, first, and of disease only secondarily. Not pity alone, but prevention foremost; not only the amelioration but the reduction of suffering was now typified in the personality of this woman not only as a possibility, but a positive policy for future generations.[8]

While applauding the cognitive aspects of motivation that were being recognized as the impetus for scientific nursing, Nutting and Dock affirmed that cognitive motivation to facilitate health would augment rather than replace the traditional moral aspects of motivation having to do with self-sacrifice, charity, and pity.

Nightingale, in her *Notes on Nursing* (1859), alluded to the association between moral and cognitive aspects of motivation. She spoke against the motivations for nursing that were accepted by society of that time, such as "disappointment in love, the want of an object, a general disgust, or incapacity for other things."[9] In addition, Nightingale also referred to benevolence and inspiration as "wild notions" for engaging in the practice of nursing.[9] It may be inferred from these references that motivation based exclusively on moral considerations was seen by Nightingale to be of as questionable a value for nursing as was motivation that developed in response to failure in other areas of life.

Nightingale added cognitive aspects of motivation to her writings by emphasizing "the laws of life and death for men" and "the laws of health for wards."[9] However, she also made references to doing God's work and bringing about the kingdom of heaven through nursing based on scientific knowledge. Nightingale thereby suggested that the cognitive aspects of motivation for caring in nursing could be employed as a means to bring about a moral good.

Moral and cognitive aspects of motivation are frequently presented in the literature as complementary rather than differentiated from each other. As an example, Bullough discussed the limitations of early nursing, when "care was motivated by a dedication to a higher cause (although) no real study of the needs of the sick had been made."[10] Bullough's study implies that a moral motivation for caring is ineffective in providing a service that is not cognitively understood.

On the other hand, writers dealing primarily with factual information on nursing often included statements that such knowledge was not complete unless accompanied by an appropriate moral-philosophic position. Nurses were directed to a "spirit of service" and an "obligation to consider others' rights as well as their own."[12,13] Heidgerken was representative of religiously oriented nursing thought in stating that "the source of supernatural motives of the Christian nurse springs from the love of God and neighbor . . . Because of her supernatural motivation, the Christian nurse will take Christ as her model."[13]

Cognitive Aspects of Motivation

Some nursing texts have directly addressed the cognitive aspects of motivation for caring by pointing out that human interrelationships are of value in themselves, and not merely the means for realizing personal moral merit or love for God.

For example, "recognition of the importance of every human being as a human being, regardless of race, religion, social or economic status" was advocated in a curriculum guide.[14]

Cognitive motivation was also alluded to by Wiedenbach, who offered three concepts basic to a philosophy of nursing: reverence for the gift of life; respect for the dignity, worth, autonomy, and individuality of each human being; and resolution to act dynamically in relation to one's beliefs.[15]

Innate Aspects of Motivation

Innate aspects of motivation are suggested in the literature through references that assign nurturing characteristics to women. Robinson, in the dual role of physician and nursing historian, stated unequivocally that "biology made the female the nurse of the species."[16] Lovell has pointed out that historically there has been a consistent trend toward societally assigning nurturing roles to women.[17]

From a different perspective, Storlie also supported the traditional position that innate aspects of motivation for caring are unique to women.[18] While directing nurses to participate in social action issues, she described nursing as the professional embodiment of women's dedication to the relief of human suffering.[18]

Nurse-historians, however, have pointed out that social and economic factors have often led to female predominance in the nursing profession. Therefore, given a different economic and social climate, there would be less differentiation between male and female participation in caring activities.[10,19,20]

Self-Reporting by Nurses Regarding Motivation for Caring

There is a limited amount of self-reporting by nurses regarding their personal motivation for caring. One applicable study was done by Oleson and Whitaker, who explored the congruence between personal professional values and characteristics ascribed to the profession by students upon graduation.[21] The phrase "demonstrating care and concern for others in an immediate and tangible way" was included in the study as an attribute under the heading "stereotyped nursing ideals." While other items under this heading showed greater divergence between personal professional values and characteristics ascribed to the profession, there was almost unanimous agreement on this item by nursing students, both at time of matriculation and at time of graduation.[21]

Self-reporting by nurses regarding motivation for caring has usually been accomplished indirectly in nursing journals through letters to the editor and first-person accounts of nursing experiences. Implicit in many of these writings is the recurring theme that nurses are concerned about the well-being of patients, are willing to participate in promoting and maintaining this well-being, and are frustrated and disappointed when they are unable to give in ways that satisfy the expectations of both nurses and patients. The "burn-out syndrome" as described by Storlie is often mentioned in relation to the inability to follow through on motivation for caring.[22]

Summary

References to moral aspects of motivation for caring in nursing are found throughout the literature. The emphasis on moral motivation is particularly prominent in nursing histories written by non-nurse authors. Nursing authors, on the other hand, have often combined moral and cognitive aspects of motivation when writing about historic nurses and when writing for nursing students. Cognitive aspects of motivation are implied in more recent texts, reflecting a trend toward viewing human interrelationships as a value in themselves and not only as a means of realizing personal moral merit or demonstrating love for God. Finally, innate aspects of motivation for caring have been inferred through references that assigned characteristics of nurturing to women. However, recent writings signal a movement away from this generalization and reflect the growing interest in the interpersonal interactions of all individuals.

HISTORICAL AND PHILOSOPHIC BACKGROUND

Nursing historians have dealt indirectly with motivation for caring in nursing by tracing the development of nursing. Pavey divided the history of nursing into three periods, thereby implying differences in motivation for each period of history.[23] The era of nursing from the dawn of history to the fourth century A.D. was described by Pavey as an art that was practiced in the family setting as an integral part of living. The transition of nursing from an art to a vocation or special calling is traced to the fourth century A.D., because it was during that time that care to the poor and infirm was extended outside the family setting by religious orders in response to the growing influence and organization of Christianity. The transition was accompanied by an emphasis on religious and moral reasons for being involved in caring for others. Nursing as a vocation was in turn succeeded by nursing as a profession in the mid-nineteenth century under Nightingale's leadership. At this time, cognitive aspects of motivation were introduced in the context of the newly developing empiric nursing knowledge.

There is little historic record about early nursing. Nutting and Dock explained this as the natural tendency of historians to overlook what was "usual and homely."[8] However, Nutting and Dock drew extensively from the 1902 writings of Kropotkin in their discussion of how innate tendencies for mutual aid and support were the underlying basis for early nursing motivation.[24] They contended that humans as well as animals possess an intuition that guides "in the selection of natural remedies, until he loses or destroys this instinct by abnormal habits or by over-civilization."[24] They thus supported Nightingale's description of the purpose of nursing as "putting the patient in the best condition for nature to act upon him."[9]

Religious Background

Continuity in nursing history begins with the early Christian era. Christian beliefs not only served as motivation for caring attitudes and behaviors, but also offered opportunities for caring outside the family setting to those who had been inhibited or restricted from doing so before by reason of societal traditions.[8]

The history of the deaconess movement in Europe can be traced to the early Christian years, when the title "diakonus" was used for both men and women who were involved in the care of the poor and sick. An example is found in the New Testament in Romans 16:1, where the original word "diakonus" was later translated to "servant" in connection with Paul's commendation of Phoebe. Nutting and Dock suggested that "while not so translated in any other connection, (it) attests probably a reluctance on the part of the translators to admit the equality of women and men in the early chuch."[7]

The transition of the diaconate of the early church to the monastic movement came gradually through the first four centuries A.D. Celibacy, segregated living, identifying apparel, and poverty vows were adopted in response to religious, social, and economic changes that occurred during that time. Along with these changes came an emphasis on the unusual and unique aspects of motivation for caring activities. Nursing came to be seen as "a penance for sins and a solace for unhappy lives."[7]

Accounts of personal commitment and devotion to caring for others during the time of monasticism indicate that such motivation and behavior were considered to be a deviation from the norm of general human involvement and possible only as the result of exceptional commitment to religious belief. It was also implied that this motivation must be independent of material considerations and monetary compensation in order to qualify as pleasing to God.

Religious teachings that emphasize doing good to others have continued to be recognized as a primary source of motivation for caring. Several different views can be identified in the context of religious motivation: (1) that love and devotion to God are primarily expressed through caring for others, (2) that caring for others is mandated by God and serves as a means of testing or proving merit, and (3) that love and devotion to God result in a unique way of viewing the world which facilitates an interest in caring about others.

While religious motivation has served as an important stimulus for concern about the well-being of others, difficulties and limitations can be found in the sense of elitism that is inherent in the idea that concern for others is not a natural human characteristic. Kropotkin referred to the distortions that he observed as religious charitable organizations translated the basic human mutual-aid tendency into charity "which bears a character of inspiration from above, and, accordingly, implies a certain superiority of the giver upon the receiver."[24]

Trilling suggested that such a sense of superiority could lead to further untoward effects, in that some paradox in our nature "leads us, when once we have made our fellow-men the objects of our enlightened interest, to go on to make the objects of our pity, then our wisdom, ultimately of our coercion."[25]

The term "prisoners of benevolence" was used by Glasser to describe the social arrangement that may develop when benefactors are recognized as superior and beneficiaries are viewed as inferior.[26] However, most religious beliefs have provided some organized attention to the caring concerns of society. Such continuity in recognizing and valuing the caring aspects of life has persisted despite strong political and economic forces that have exerted influence in favor of competition and rivalry.

Political and Economic Influences

The theology of the medieval period continues to be a pervasive part of our philosophic ideologies, according to McLaughlin.[27]

Two main religious and societal beliefs became integrated in a way that has significantly influenced economic and political thought: (1) In the context of religious ideations regarding motivation, it was inappropriate to associate payment with caring services; and (2) according to general societal understanding, women were assigned to be primary caregivers by reason of natural order.

Out of such societally accepted standards, economic and political policies were developed that opposed the recognition and reward of caring services. Saiving has pointed out that caring activities came to be devalued in comparison with more aggressive and external achievements.[28]

Osborne found that a survey of philosophic literature on women's issues revealed a general trend toward defining women by their caring roles as well as minimizing the importance of caring.[29]

An example of this trend can be seen in Rousseau's explanation that the role of women in caring is determined by natural order:

> That obedience which she owes her husband, that care and tenderness which is due to her children, are such natural and affecting consequences of her situation, that unless she is abandoned to a habitual depravity, she cannot revolt from those internal principles which influence her conduct; nor mistake her duty, while she retains that propensity which nature has implanted in her bosom.[29]

Another influential philosopher, Kant, described women as having innate characteristics of "many sympathetic feelings, much goodheartedness and compassion," and claimed that "Providence hath implanted in their breasts humane and benevolent sentiments" which are not expected to be found naturally in men.[29]

Schopenhauer contended that women show more sympathy for the unfortunate than do men because they are by nature inferior to men in point of justice.[29] Nietzsche reiterated this belief and extended it with the notion that the movement for equality for women would result in women losing their nature and instincts, which were their only redeeming traits.[29]

On the other hand, Mills spoke out against the subjection of women. He believed that women had innate tendencies that were necessary to society for "fostering the sentiments and continuing the traditions of spirit and generosity."[29] Paradoxically, however, he contended that this tendency, although innate, could not be effectively utilized without the reinforcement of education, which would direct the thoughts and purposes of women into fields of service.[29]

Gould analyzed the writings of philosophers regarding sex-linked characteristics of morals and values, and found that writers often allowed their views on universal human nature to be influenced by the cultural prejudices of their time.[30] Gould further pointed out that it is not because women have been considered to be of secondary importance that their caring traits have been labeled as secondary. Rather, she argues that because women have had a subordinate role in society, and because traits of aesthetic sensitivity, intuition, and caring have also been of secondary importance, therefore, these traits have been assigned to women as feminine characteristics.

> On this hypothesis it can be seen that the assignment of "male" and "female" characteristics as respectively dominant or subordinate, or essential or accidental, is a product of contingent priorities at a given historical stage of social and political development.[30]

According to Marnel, it is a reliable phenomenon of human nature that as ideas pass, they are passed down.[31] The passing down of incomplete and outdated philosophies of motivation for caring has resulted in contradictory perceptions regarding the values placed on caring within the nursing profession as well as within the larger society. Ashley pointed out that our understanding of caring in nursing has been curtailed and limited through philosophic and historic traditions as they have been passed down through the closed systems of hospitals and nursing schools.[19] The hierarchic structure of the hospital, with its rigid status symbols and its inadequate channels of communication, has not gone through liberating changes at the same rate as the rest of society.[32]

Humanistic Influences

In humanism, it is not considered necessary to look to supernatural explanations for a motivation for caring. Instead, the humanistic ethic is focused on the cognitive process of understanding the empiric laws that underlie human relationships. The supreme good is conceived as the object that satisfies all individuals.[32] The intent of humanism is to address the joint and inclusive satisfaction of all individuals, seeing human beings as ends in themselves and not merely as means. However, distortions may arise if the good of others comes to be seen as the means for producing good for oneself, thereby resulting in the tendency to dictate to others to what good they must aspire. Anderson contended that the approach to public policy must be fundamentally different in the humanistic ethic.[34] The purpose is not to remove a potential source of crime, "or even to make certain individuals more 'socially productive,' but rather to release the fullest possibilities of human development."[34]

Anderson pointed out that humanistic policies are unfamiliar to our society and therefore may be difficult to implement consistently. However, the cognitive aspects of motivation that are found in the humanistic movement can lead to a renewed understanding of the innate human aspects of motivation for caring. As Blanchette stated,

> any attempt to describe the struggle of history only in terms of animosity between classes, races or any other sort of human grouping is not only an oversimplification, but it is a reduction of what is most internal in the struggle to what is purely external and it is an oversight of what is most essential, the desire for communion that is at the source of the struggle itself.[35]

There is increased interest in the biologic tendencies that influence human interactions. The traditional view that innate caring characteristics are predominantly feminine is being replaced with the understanding that both sexes have the capacity for caring behaviors.[36],[37]

Attention is also being focused on the mutual-aid tendencies of our species, as first advanced by Kropotkin in rebuttal of aspects of Darwinian theory.

> The mutual-aid tendency in man has so remote an origin, and is so deeply interwoven with all the past evolution of the human race, that it has been maintained by mankind up to the present time, notwithstanding all vicissitudes of history . . . . The ethical progress of our race, viewed in its broad lines, appears as a gradual extension of the mutual-aid principles from the tribe to always larger and larger agglomerations, so as to finally embrace one day the whole of mankind, without respect to its diverse creeds, languages and races.[34]

Kropotkin's optimistic view regarding innate human caring characteristics is tempered by present sociobiologic views that see "seemingly altruistic acts bestowed on tribe and nation, directed, sometimes very circuitously, toward the Darwinian advantage of the solitary human being and his closest relatives."[38]

Whether from Kropotkin's view that man's innate tendencies to do good need only be freed from the restrictions placed on them by political and economic forces, or from Wilson's view that cultural evolution of higher ethical values cannot replace or exceed genetic evolution, the growing interest in the innate aspects of motivation for caring is of significance to the nursing profession, which has been developed around the idea of caring roles and services.

Implications for Nursing Practice

Our present understanding of the appropriate motivation for caring continues to be influenced by the historic and philosophic background of our society. Notions that caring requires exceptional motivation and does not command commensurate reward have come down to us from past religious belief systems. These beliefs have been integrated with other notions regarding the secondary importance of women and caring attitudes and behaviors in our society. Together, these ideas have been incorporated into our beliefs and values and have posed a barrier to the full development of the profession of nursing, which has been organized around caring roles and services.

Nurses living within the nursing culture as well as within the broader realm of society frequently experience frustration and confusion as contradictions are encountered between the various aspects of personal and professional life. A dilemma arises from their occupying a fundamental role in society while occupying a marginal role in economic and political life, as pointed out by Mitchell.[39]

Caring in nursing has a fundamental role in promoting the well-being of our society, yet has remained on the periphery of economic and political decision-making. In the context of fundamental versus marginal role differences, along with religious and sexist misconceptions regarding the motivation for caring, it has been difficult for the nursing profession to maintain a clear understanding of the relationship between the concept of caring and the practice of nursing.

Awareness of historic forces that have made an impact on our present perceptions about appropriate motivation for caring in nursing can be helpful when analyzing issues about which there is conflict in nursing education and practice. There is a need to recognize our residual societal perceptions that caring is a result of exceptional motivation equivalent to a religious vocation, or that it is primarily a feminine trait that is of secondary importance. Such notions have persisted because it has been difficult to separate them out for critical scrutiny, interwoven as they are with our valued institutions of church and family.

Objective analysis of motivation for caring in nursing can lead to a clearer perspective of the concept of caring as a significant universal human capacity as well as an intentioned, proficient, professional service in nursing.

REFERENCES

1. Leininger M: Caring: An Essential Human Need. Thorofare, NJ, Charles B. Slack Inc., 1981.
2. Leininger M: Transcultural Nursing: Concepts, Theories and Practice. New York, John Wiley & Sons, 1978.
3. Watson J: Nursing: The Philosophy and Science of Caring. Boston, Little, Brown and Co., 1979.
4. Dickoff J, James P: Beliefs and values: bases for curriculum design. Nursing Research 17(5):415–427, 1970.
5. Titmuss RM: The Gift Relationship: From Human Blood to Social Policy. New York, Pantheon Books, 1971.
6. Saunders L: Permanence and change. In Lewis EP: Changing Patterns of Nursing Practice. New York, The American Journal of Nursing Company, 1971.
7. Nutting MA, Dock LL: A History of Nursing, Volume II. New York, Putnam, 1935, pp 75, 100–104.
8. Nutting MA, Dock LL: A History of Nursing, Volume II. New York, Putnam, 1935, pp 17, 99, 134.
9. Nightingale F: Notes on Nursing: What It Is, and What It Is Not. London, Lippincott, 1946, p 75.
10. Bullough B: The Emergence of Modern Nursing, 2nd ed. New York, Macmillan, 1969, p 56.
11. National League for Nursing: A Curriculum for Schools of Nursing. New York, National League for Nursing, 1932, pp 36–37.
12. Stewart IM: The Education of Nurses. New York, Macmillan, 1943, p 307.
13. Heidgerken LE: Teaching and Learning in Schools of Nursing. Philadelphia, PA, JB Lippincott Co., 1965, p 88.
14. Sand O: Curriculum Study in Basic Nursing Education. New York, Putnam, 1955, p 43.
15. Wiedenbach E: Clinical Nursing, A Helping Art. New York, Springer Publishing, 1964, p 16.
16. Robinson V: White Caps, The Story of Nursing. Philadelphia, PA, JB Lippincott Co., 1946, p 360.
17. Lovell MC: Silent but perfect partners: medicine's use and abuse of women. Advances in Nursing Science 3(2):25–40, 1981.
18. Storlie F: Nursing and the Social Conscience. New York, Appleton, Century-Crofts, 1970, p 2.

19. Ashley J: Hospitals, Paternalism, and the Role of the Nurse. New York, Teachers College Press, 1976.
20. Dolan JA: Nursing in Society, 14th ed. Philadelphia, PA, WB Saunders Co., 1979.
21. Oleson V, Whitaker E: The Silent Dialogue. San Francisco, CA, Jossey Bass, 1968, pp 123–131.
22. Storlie F: Burnout: the elaboration of a concept. Nursing 79(12):2108–2111, 1979.
23. Pavey AE: The Story of the Growth of Nursing. Philadelphia, PA, JB Lippincott Co., 1953.
24. Kropotkin P: Mutual Aid. New York, Garland Publishing, 1972, pp 11, 223, 283.
25. Trilling L: The Liberal Imagination. Garden City, NY, Anchor Books, Doubleday, 1950, p 215.
26. Gaylin W: Doing Good, The Limits of Benevolence. New York, Pantheon Books, 1978, pp 97–108.
27. McLaughlin E: Equality of souls, inequality of sexes: women in western thought. *In* Osborne ML (ed): Women in Western Thought. New York, Random House, 1979.
28. Saiving V: The human situation: a feminine view. *In* Christ CP, Plaskow J: Womenspirit Rising. San Francisco, CA, Harper and Row, 1979, p 35.
29. Osborne ML (ed): Women in Western Thought. New York, Random House, 1979, pp 11, 155, 214, 272.
30. Gould CC: Women and Philosophy: Toward a Theory of Liberation. New York, Putnam, 1976, pp 22–23.
31. Marnel WH: Man-Made Morals, Four Philosophies That Shaped America. New York, Doubleday, 1965, p 256.
32. Brown EL: Newer Dimensions of Patient Care. New York, Little, Brown, 1961, p 22.
33. Bierman AK: Life and Morals. New York, Harcourt Brace Jovanovich, 190, p 390.
34. Anderson W: Politics and the New Humanism. Pacific Palisades, CA, Goodyear Publishing, 1973, p 144.
35. Blanchette O: For a Fundamental Social Ethic—A Philosophy of Social Change. New York, Philosophical Library, 1973, p 140.
36. Gaylin W: Caring. New York, Avon Books, 1976.
37. Meyeroff M: On Caring. New York, Perennial Library, 1971.
38. Wilson EO: On Human Nature. New York, Bantam Books, 1978, p 165.
39. Mitchell J: Social structure and sexual oppression. *In* Bierman AK, Gould JA (eds): Philosophy for a New Generation. New York, Macmillan, 1977, p 466.

6

Themes and Issues in Conceptualizing Care

The purpose of this chapter is to address issues and themes emerging in the current research on care. The assumption that care is a culturally relevant domain that organizes human experience has prompted the research of a small group of nurses and anthropologists for the past decade. Leininger first made explicit the link between nursing, care, and cross-cultural variation.[1,2] Her contribution to the nursing theory of the concept of care is akin to the development of a new paradigm, as characterized by Kuhn.[3] If we accept this analogy, it remains for the rest of us to define further, refine, and develop the concept of care.[1]

Nursing has yet to confront the full potential of caregiving as a human response and a functioning component of a health and healing system. The nature of care and the variations in cultural content of care behavior continue to appear illusive, amorphous, and ambiguous; yet cultural patterns for "taking care of self" and "taking care of others" provide explanations for all manner of human behavior. When early man first developed into a symbolizing, upright creature, the experience of discomfort and well-being, of itching and nonitching, of fatigue and nonfatigue created conditions to be explained and understood, as well as settings requiring culturally constructed ways of behaving.

This chapter addresses the following themes: (1) Care as a culturally relevant domain; (2) care as a central concept of nursing; and (3) ways of making the dimensions of the care an explicit concept.

CARE AS A CULTURALLY RELEVANT DOMAIN

With the exception of Leininger's work, care has received scant attention in the anthropologic literature. Nurture, helping behaviors, and child and sibling caretaking—as described in the works of Whiting, Weisner, Gallimore, and Honigmann—are examples of ethnographic findings that treat care as a social situation containing actors who know, or are learning ways to be accountable for, what happens to human beings, objects, or events.[4-6]

In an earlier paper, the author attempted to delineate principles of heuristic value for the study of care based on the following themes: searching for universals, fitting within a cultural system, using the developmental process, and cultural variations in form.[7] For example, two societies now extinct—the Ik and the Mundugumor—give anthropologists examples of societies in which it is uncertain whether care is valued, takes a unique form of expression, or is not manifest at all. This raises the question of whether there is a universal expression of care in different cultures.[8,9]

A second theme useful to the study of care is how it fits into a cultural health and healing system. In the anthropologic literature, it is clear that all cultures provide explanations for the inevitable experiences of birth, disease, and death. How these explanations fit within the system continue to be of interest to nurse anthropologists, medical anthropologists, and so on. Belief in that which is imbued with power is a central focus for the study of health and healing systems.[10] Most work attends to causes of illness and health, rituals of professionals, and use of drugs. Little attention is directed at the illusive characteristics of doing things for others or self and how these events fit within a cultural system. We know about exchanges among individuals in receiving or giving care, that is, rubbing a back, washing and dressing a *santo*, and being attended to when one is sick in bed with a dripping nose and multiple bodily aches and pains. Knowing how the meaning of these events is linked within a cultural system can add to our understanding of care. Information on the context or "fit" within specific systems adds to what we know about conceptualizations of care—the core as well as the boundaries of the concept.

The developmental process provides a third dimension for conceptualizing care. Changes in beliefs and values during the life cycle of individuals, families, and societies tell us about attributes of care that change through time. For example, the author's work on the child's view of health and healing provided beginning data on changes in food exchange, teaching, monitoring the well-being and comfort of others, and controlling one's thoughts.[11] Examples of caregiving during mother-child interactions include a five-year-old who wakes his mother and then lets her sleep ten minutes longer, and a four-year-old girl with a recipe for a stomach ache—that is, lying prone on your stomach and pressing hard.

Finally, diversity in speech or cultural variations in form help us to comprehend differences among cultural groups. For example, studying the variation between participants in a popular culture of caregiving (ie, neighbors, family members, students) and professional health caretakers can add to our understanding. Neighbors exchange chores, check on each other, and watch out for burglars. Family scenes provide time and space for touching and talking out feelings. Students confide in each other when they are "down," and go for walks, lend money, and tell jokes. Professional caregivers, on the other hand, monitor life-support systems, lift heads to reach the lip of a glass of water, scratch a toe for someone in a full body cast, and talk with patients and families. Such diversity and variation in the cultural forms of care, caregiving, and caring suggest that there exist wide-ranging patterns of behavior that assist in organizing human experience during social interaction.

CARE: THE CENTRAL CONCEPT OF NURSING

Since the time of Florence Nightingale, the nurse has been expected to serve as the prime practitioner of care. Nightingale wrote that the goal for nursing is "to put the patient(s) in the best condition for nature to act" upon them. [12] Despite the approximately 125 years during which nursing has recognized this charter, the idea or concept of care remains vague, ambiguous, and often invisible when cost-accounting for nursing services is done. In one sense, care is cheap— that is, everyone, with either great or little skill, can do it. Care has also been surrounded with connotations of sweetness, emotionality, and doing for others. If care were a limited good such as jewels (diamonds, emeralds) or natural resources (coal, oil, gas), we probably would have a better grasp of the concept, and it would have greater economic value. Nevertheless, nursing must make explicit at all levels of analysis what care is about.

WAYS TO MAKE CARE EXPLICIT

The work of Leininger has led to the identification of 40 ethnocaring and nursing care constructs, ie, comfort, empathy, succor, surveillance, and tenderness, among others. [13,14] These constructs have emerged in her analysis of data from 30 cultures. A major theme in her writing is that each culture is taught a different system of patterning derived from various sets of these constructs and from the people's viewpoint and their meanings of care. This is a major contribution to the science of care.

Using a somewhat similar method, at the University of Arizona we have generated a beginning list of constructs with primitive meanings. These constructs or meanings have emerged in studies directed at understanding the cultural knowledge that is used as human beings care for others or for themselves. From 15 studies conducted in different social situations, in both professional and popular contexts, we have collected ethnographic data illustrating the native's view of caregiving, as well as the researcher's view of the native's view. Following the protocol of Spradley, we have used participant observation and ethnographic interviews to generate domains of meaning and a taxonomic structure within each meaning. [15,16] Additionally, from the ethnographic data, we have used Spradley's ideas (from the work of Opler) about the cultural theme to generate conceptualizations representing the whole of the cultural patterning from the researcher's view. [17]

Studies have focused on clients in hospital settings, family members, teenagers, Norwegian-Americans, children with alopecia (hair loss), mothers and fathers monitoring health care of children, the elderly in ambulatory health care settings, and interactions between mothers and preschoolers. In the approximately 15 studies, we have uncovered 20 cultural themes characterizing different dimensions of care, caring, and caregiving. In this analysis, we have ordered the themes according to three roles implicit in the caregiving process: caregiver or caretaker, care recipient or they-who-are-being-cared-for, and care of self or self-care. In each study, the focus of the ethnographic data was the native's view. The following individuals organized their experience using, at one time or another, each of these dimensions of giver, receiver, or self-carer: the native as a child, a clinic patient, a member of a society, a neighbor, a child undergoing a painful procedure, a father of a sick child, or a family member in a waiting room. Assignment of the data to one or another dimension then depended on the role best represented by the native in the view of the researcher.

CAREGIVER ROLE

Domains of meaning and informing behavior in the role of caregiver were: Be there; Stay close; Stay cool (don't be hysterical, do not draw attention); Treat me as normal; Get a good doctor; Talk about the future and past, not the present; Let me participate in my care; Fix the coffee. This cognitive ordering is not unfamiliar to any health care provider. Implicit in these meanings are the rules for presenting oneself, for ordering the ritualistic activity (ie, get a good doctor and make coffee), and for recognizing the participation of the receiver. In our data, we are only beginning to hear about overload of caregiving or domains such as "leave me alone sometimes," and joking behavior associated with exchanging caretaking. The real world tells us that the caregiving role is more complicated than we are yet able to portray.

RECEIVER OF CARE

The rules for receiving care are implied in the domains: The nurses don't come for things; The pits of dependency is not being able to scratch yourself; I wish I could, but you won't let me; I can't do it on my own, but I want to; Be strong and in control; Learning how to receive care is possible; It's important that someone really cares, even for a few minutes. We know less about the role of dependency or being the receiver of care. These domains of meaning suggest that there are more aspects than in caregiving, that there are good and bad things to have done for you, and that role conflict is a complex issue.

SELF-CARE

Domains of meaning in self-care focus on setting the stage for what has been, is, or is about to be; on talking to oneself; and on using strategies for staying cool and in control. They are: The importance of knowing; The stroke may come any minute; Control yourself or what you have will control you; Get used to it or work on acceptance; Things to do for hurting (for example: moan, tighten up muscles, say "The Lord is my Shepherd," count numbers, squeeze Dad's thumb); How I think makes a difference (self-hypnosis); and Try not to move.

To date, our ethnographic data are showing us some of the diversity that can contribute to our understanding of the complexities in conceptualizations of care. There is much work to do. We continue to ask the questions: What can the cultural concept contribute to our understanding of care? Must a study of care be grounded in culture? For us, this is so, but for other disciplines the world is different. The question of how biologic variables meet with behavioral variables in a construct of care or caregiving is yet a mystery. The concept of care represents the real work of nursing. The obligation for nursing is to understand how care is performed throughout the human and animal world.

REFERENCES

1. Leininger M: Nursing and Anthropology: Two Worlds to Blend. New York, John Wiley & Sons, 1970.
2. Leininger M: Convergence and divergence of human behavior: an ethnopsychological comparative study of two Gadsup villages in the eastern highlands of New Guinea. Doctoral, University of Washington, 1966.
3. Kuhn T: The Structure of Scientific Revolutions. Chicago, IL, The University of Chicago Press, 1962.
4. Whiting J: Field Guide for Study of Socialization. New York, John Wiley & Sons, 1966.
5. Weisner TS, Gallimore R: My brother's keeper: child and sibling caretaking. Current Anthropology 18(2):169-190, 1977.
6. Honigmann JJ: Responsibility and nurturance: an Austrian example. J Psychol Anthropol 1(1):81-100, 1978.
7. Aamodt A: The care component in a health and healing system. In Bauwens E(ed): Anthropology and Health. St. Louis, MO, C.V. Mosby, 1978, pp 37-45.
8. Turnbull C: The Mountain People. New York, Simon and Schuster, 1972.
9. Mead M: Male and Female. New York, New American Library of World Literature, Inc., 1949.
10. Glick LB: Medicine as an ethnographic category: the Zioni of the New Guinea highlands. Ethnology 6:31-55, 1967.
11. Aamodt M: The child's view of health and healing. Communicating Nursing Research 5:38-54, 1972.
12. Nightingale F: Notes on Nursing. New York, Appleton-Century-Crofts, 1859.
13. Leininger M: Transcultural Nursing: Concepts, Theories and Practices. New York, John Wiley & Sons, 1978.
14. Leininger M: Caring: An Essential Human Need. Thorofare, NJ, Charles B. Slack, Inc., 1981.
15. Spradley J: The Ethnographic Interview. New York, Holt, Rinehart and Winston, 1979.
16. Spradley J: Participant Observation. New York, Holt, Rinehart and Winston, 1980.

PART TWO: Research and Application to Nursing

7

Caring is Nursing: Understanding the Meaning, Importance, and Issues

Every discipline tends to use special terms and expressions to communicate the distinctive features, areas of interest, or attributes of the field. Such practices help one to recognize the discipline and the expected domains of knowledge. Common language usage in any culture binds not only disciplines but also people together for a variety of reasons.

In the field of nursing, the author holds that the linguistic term and concomitant phrases related to care and nursing care have special meanings and patterns of usage that are often not fully recognized and understood by the nursing profession. "Care" and "nursing care" are taken for granted as expressions, almost like saying "good morning" and "hello." However, the author contends that "care" or "caring" is one of nursing's unique terms, and it has many special and diverse meanings for nurses and clients.

Caring is nursing, and nursing is caring.[1] Caring is the linguistic term that communicates to others nursing's unique and unifying focus. Caring makes nursing understandable to those who have known and experienced care from nurses in diverse ways. Caring is nursing's unique contribution to society and to its evolving discipline. Caring is the unique, unifying, and dominant focus of nursing.[2,3]

The abovementioned statements are full of assumptions and philosophic, theoretic, and experiential ideas. Since the mid-1950s, the author has promoted and encouraged care as the area that offers the most promise for establishing a body of substantive knowledge in nursing. However, the response of nurses has been slow, since they tend to take for granted that which they purport to know from a microperspective. Some nurses tend to devalue and demean the concept of care. What care means to nurses and how care is operationalized and used to help people remain true enigmas and a domain of inquiry.

This chapter addresses some pertinent issues, questions, and thoughts about care. The linguistic uses of care in the profession, factors influencing the systematic study of care, and the transmission of care in teaching and practice are highlighted.

Nurses have used care as a mode of thought, action, and language for nearly a century. Then what makes care so difficult to study or to promote for its scientific, historic, and humanistic meanings? Only in the past decade have a few nurses begun to explore the multiple meanings and usages in the profession through National Caring Conferences.[3] It is a curious fact that nurse-researchers tend to study phenomena such as health, energy, human environment, coping, rhythms, time, and other similar concepts, but leave care, on the whole, unexplored. At the same time, however, nurses make verbal and active claims to care as caregivers or providers. There is an obvious gap between nurses' claims and their research interests. Interestingly, the public tends to emphasize care as nursing's art and skill, and some citizens have contributed money to have nurses study care. Such paradoxic behavior makes one realize the need to study and understand nurses' behaviors and care phenomena. The potential to explicate care and to make it the philosophic and practical base of nursing appears evident. Care remains largely the "sleeper construct" yet to be discovered through in-depth systematic investigations.

In several publications, the author has stated that *care* is the *central, dominant, and unifying focus of nursing*.[3,4] She holds that the construct of care is of major importance to nursing and must be systematically studied to make known the full nature and manifestations of care, nursing care, and related behaviors and processes. There are many ideas and practices that can be identified with care as nurses engage in caring activities. Accordingly, nurses need to communicate their care services to the public. Providing different care to people from diverse cultures could well lead to a major breakthrough in nursing and the health fields. Such challenges and potentials make us realize that care remains the most promising and exciting construct to be fully discovered in nursing and the health fields.

A HISTORIC NOTE

Shortly after the author established the field of transcultural nursing in the mid-1950s as a legitimate and formal area of study and practice, the critical need to focus on care phenomena from a transcultural nursing perspective became apparent. Transcultural nursing as *comparative caring* was defined as follows: an area of study and practice focusing upon the differences and similarities among cultures with respect to health and illness caring values, practices, and beliefs in order to provide culture-specific or cultural-universal nursing care to people.[5] As a consequence, care was central to transcultural nursing and an area of study for all aspects of nursing.

This leads to the idea of establishing care as nursing's major philosophic, theoretic, and clinical area of scientific and humanistic study. Care could be a distinct, unifying, and major area of practice if nurse-researchers would study patterns and themes of care in different cultures and environmental settings. Understanding care in its biophysical, social, political, and cultural dimensions is needed.

An anthropologic perspective of holistic generic man, along with transcultural nursing research, could lead to universal principles and laws about nursing care in different human contexts. The idea of care as being culturally constituted and expressed was entirely new to most nurses. Hence, considerable education from an anthropologic perspective was needed, as well as preparation of a cadre of nurse-anthropologists to lay the groundwork for transcultural care. The 1960s and 1970s were devoted to the preparation of nurses by means of five or six years of study—in cultural, physical, and social anthropology. An effort to retain interest in comparative care from both a nursing and an anthropologic viewpoint was also made.

From her own studies, the author hypothesized that care was an essential human need for birth, growth, survival, and for people who are dying. Both a nursing and an anthropologic viewpoint is important to grasping the role of care and care activities throughout time and in many cultures. Care appeared essential, in the anthropologic record, to human survival and development.

In the early 1960s, the author conducted the first transcultural *emic* study of care in a non-Western culture, the Eastern Highlands of New Guinea.[6] She discovered that cultures could identify, define, and discuss the meaning of care, and that care was not only in a professional nurse's repertoire. Since then, she has studied five major cultures intensively, and 25 cultures through ethnographic literature and other ethnonursing research methods.[6] In the mid-1970s, she launched the National Research Caring Conferences. At these national meetings, several theoretic, philosophic, and research works by nurses specializing in care have been presented to explicate the phenomenon of care. This national meeting and the National Transcultural Nursing Conferences are the only ones in nursing focused per se on care phenomena. Progress is being made, with encouraging outcomes. It is important to note this is the second program focused on the care phenomenon held at the American Nurses Association convention. (The first program was also spearheaded by the author in 1976.) It appears that our national professional nursing organizations have had limited interest in the phenomenon of care and in supporting care as a major domain of nursing. The author believes, however, that sooner or later nurse leaders will awaken to the importance of care and will support the concept in research and teaching. It is of interest to find that nursing students are generally the strongest supporters of care, except for the group of care researchers.

Gaut, a nurse philosopher and active care researcher, found that nurses used care as a slogan or as an ambiguous word with limited meanings.[7] She states: "But what is it about caring that makes it so usable? Is it a concept through which practices and policies can be justified, or is it a vague and ambiguous term . . ."[7] Her findings corroborate the author's in that she found that nurses use the term without much thought about its meaning and usage in different nursing contexts. Some nurses use care as if it were a magical word and one that brings magical outcomes. For example, nurses say: "I gave him care and he is doing fine"; "I cared for her and she will get well." Gaut's position that care has limited philosophic meaning as a slogan or an expression merits attention by nurses.

It is interesting that with the present cultural movement to emphasize and study care, there are now more nurses, physicians, social workers, and others using the word "care," but in different ways.[1] Care seems to be a popular word, but its diverse meanings remain obscure. When asked, some nurses say: "By care, I mean protection"; others will say, "I mean care and nothing else." Observing clients' responses to the actions of nurses is an important way to study care. It is also interesting to study noncaring perceptions of nurses and clients to determine what constitutes care. Nurses committed to medical regimens seldom use the term "care," but rather speak of tasks to be done.

To date, "care" has had multiple professional, popular, and social usages and meanings. Professional and nonprofessional views of care can be identified as well as caring and noncaring behaviors on the parts of nurses. The value and importance of care and the potential for establishing a body of knowledge related to it have yet to be discovered on a national and international basis. Currently, only a small percentage of nurses (estimated to be less than 10%) are systematically investigating and promoting care research.

DEFINITION OF TERMS

The following definitions are used in this paper:[1]

Care/caring: refers, in a generic sense, to those assistive, supportive, or facilitative acts toward or for another individual or group with evident or anticipated needs, to ameliorate or improve a human condition or lifeway.

Professional nursing care: those cognitively learned humanistic and scientific modes of helping or enabling an individual, family, or community to receive personalized services through culturally specific or ascribed caring processes, techniques, and patterns in order to improve or maintain a favorably healthy condition for life or death.

WHY THE DELAY IN FOCUSING ON CARE

It is an interesting paradox to consider why nurses have delayed studying care phenomena. On the one hand, nurses continue to claim to be caregivers. On the other hand, nurses are not systematically investigating care as the central and dominant construct of nursing. From the author's study and observations, there are several factors that might clarify such behaviors.

1. Nurses who practice care tend to believe that they know all about care, and have limited interest in looking at care in depth. As one nurse said, "I have

practiced care daily in my work, I know all about it." When asked further about the meaning and characteristics of care, she replied: "I really have not thought about those aspects of care. I just give it." This action view of care without examination of its nature, meaning, and distinguishable features tends to be common among action-oriented caregivers.

2. The lack of nurse-researchers studying the philosophic and epistemologic aspects of care, as well as its effects, has greatly curtailed work on the phenomenon. Other theoretic and conceptual ideas seem to take precedence over care for nurses; for example, energy flow, medical symptoms, and disease. Concepts such as empathy, love, compassion, presence, and other care constructs probably appear to be more difficult to study and more difficult to measure or know in a comprehensive way. Nurses who have studied the liberal arts and humanities, anthropology, and philosophy tend to be more interested in care and the ideas comprising its major construct.

3. Myths and slogans about care have prevailed in nursing, such as the following: "Cure is more important than care." "Doing technical tasks and medical activities is what clients want when they are ill." "Care is too difficult to study and understand." "There's not time to give or practice care." "What the physician says and does is mainly what counts." It is also believed that Florence Nightingale wrote all about care and defined it. In reality, Nightingale did not define, explicate, or study care phenomena per se. In her *Notes on Nursing*, Nightingale speaks indirectly about carelike conditions such as the need for air, food, ventilation, and proper environment, and about putting the patient in the proper environment for nature to help him.[8] If Nightingale were living today, she would undoubtedly be pleased to know that some nurses are focusing on care and different environments in which to help clients.

4. The rapid developments in technology since World War II have been another factor delaying the study of care, in that nurses have become actively involved with many technologic devices and procedures. While there are different types of technologic care, there are still many other kinds of care that have not been explored, such as interpersonal, political, cultural, social, and religious care. As technologic services increase, one can predict that there will be less time for other kinds of care services such as providing comfort measures, offering personalized support, and being present when the client needs solace.

5. The dominant emphasis on medical *curing* techniques, diagnoses, and treatment has decreased nurses' interest in studying care as an important or worthwhile phenomenon. Conceptualizing nursing as medical tasks

and activities rather than explicit care activities, decision, and thoughts has had its impact on advancing knowledge about care. The power of physicians to cure and to get public support for such actions has not been an incentive to study care. As a consequence, nonmedical and nontechnical care has been studied limitedly. Nurses caught up in medical curing processes tend to devalue care activities and the study and practice of care.

6. Until recently, care was largely perceived by female nurses as "too feminine" and an activity of less status than curing. Hence, some nurses wanted to dissociate themselves from care. This is one reason why they do not like to focus on care; they focus on cure, realizing that cure tends to dominate as a medical value. Anthropologically speaking, males can and do care for others, and it can denote status. The connotation of care as uniquely female is maintained by feminism but cannot be supported. It appears that nurses' need for status and recognition, and their fear of being demeaned while caring for others, can explain part of their behavior related to care. Accordingly, some nursing professors expressed concern about emphasizing care because of their negative feelings about care as a female activity. Such traditional viewpoints need to be reexamined, since care has long been an altruistic, noble, and recognized value in several cultures throughout history. In fact, male health care providers often envy female caregivers and their healing powers. Thus, negative myths about sex-linked roles appear to limit nurses' interest in studying and providing care.

7. Care has not been systematically studied until recently because qualitative research methods have been only limitedly valued in nursing, and care research generally necessitates knowledge and skills related to qualitative methods. Currently, in graduate programs there is much emphasis on quantitative research methods. Searching for the meaning of care and identifying its attributes require skill in the use of qualitative methods. While one may wish to measure care, there are other features that are nonmeasurable or not reducible to numbers. The participant-observation and ethnonursing research methods are just beginning to receive attention in nursing, and are opening the door to explicating and understanding obscure facets of care. The past absence of documentation of details and processes by nurses has also limited the investigation of care.

8. There are very few nurses prepared in the use of historic research methods or in cultural historic processes, which has handicapped nurses in knowing and valuing care with respect to different cultures in the world. Transcultural nurses have been active in discovering aspects of care from anthropologic and nursing data, but much more work lies ahead before the prehistory and history of nursing and care are known. How care

services have contributed to human survival for millions of years is an important topic to address. Nurse anthropologists know that care must have existed throughout history for the human species to have survived millions of years. The author believes that nurses with an anthropologic and transcultural nursing background will be able to identify care features and their actual or predicted effect on human cultures in the future. Transcultural nurses remain the major group to study the historic and prehistoric aspects of care.

9. The lack of theories about care until recently also limited the development of scientific and humanistic knowledge about care. Currently, the author's theory of transcultural care is providing the major focus for care studies in nursing. The variability and universality of care and especially of its components, such as trust, compassion, support, nurture, comfort, presence, and others, remain open to transcultural theoretic studies. While Orem's theory of self-care is promising for explicating one aspect of care, it is culture bound and fails to recognize cross-cultural manifestations and other care modalities.[9]

10. Another factor that appears to have delayed the study of care has been the lack of emphasis by the American Nurses Association, the National League for Nursing, the American Association of Colleges of Nursing, and other nursing organizations. Accordingly, there has been virtually no *research money* to study care supplied by these national nursing organizations. There have also been no explicit funds from federal and state nursing agencies to support care studies per se. It is hoped that this will occur before the end of this decade.

11. Last but not least, there has been limited *economic value* placed on care by hospital administrators, physicians, and other health agencies providing monies for health care. Ray's study highlights the absence of economic support for care, but reveals that technologic care and medical diagnostic activities receive economic sanctions and awards.[10] Until nurses and others place a high economic value on care, it will be difficult to get funds. Economic value must be linked to nursing care that listens to clients, provides comfort measures, or provides other forms of care services.

CONCEPTUAL MODEL AND THEORY OF CARE STUDY

In several publications, the author has already presented her conceptual model, hypotheses, assumptions, and philosophic stance about care.[11-13] The reader is encouraged to review these sources to understand the rich potentials for investigating care. The author's theory of transcultural nursing care, with research from many cultures, has also recently been published.

Currently, there are few macro or micro conceptual models and explicit theories that focus on care phenomenon, especially from a cross-cultural viewpoint. As indicated previously, Orem's theory of self-care fails to theorize about care from cross-culture, social-structure, and world-view perspectives.[9] Orem's theory remains an Anglo-American one with Western assumptions about self-care behaviors.

In the nearly 40 cultures studied by the author, the theory of diversity and universality in cultural care from social-structure and world views has been extremely valuable in studying and documenting differential care perspectives, expressions, and actions of cultures regarding care. The author's macro-model and theory continue to guide nurses in studying care and in searching for universals or specific attributes. To date, the findings about cross-cultural care reveal more differences than similarities among cultures.[14] More important, however, cultures do have cognitive perceptions, values, beliefs, and practices about care than can be documented. Functional and structural features related to care have also been identified.[12]

MAJOR ISSUES IN CARING AND NURSING CARE KNOWLEDGE AND PRACTICES

In this last section, a few specific issues related to the development of care knowledge and nursing care practices are identified. One of the important issues is whether the nursing profession will be committed to care as its dominant, central, and unifying domain. Will nurses be willing to study care as a distinct phenomenon of the discipline of nursing? The author believes that nurses need to have at least one dominant idea to help support the nature, essence, and major characteristic of nursing as a discipline and profession. To date, nursing has no central focus, only many loose and largely unverified domains of knowledge. It is conceivable that in time there may be other central domains, but care is the most obvious, most familiar, and best known by nurses. It is interesting that since the author and her colleagues began to focus on care in the past decade, other disciplines have become interested in care, ie, philosophers, physicians, child development specialists, anthropologists, and so forth. Will these disciplines develop care, with nurses reacting later, since this construct belongs historically to them? While other disciplines may study care, nurses have still had more than 100 years' experience with care and should be the leaders in the study of the care phenomenon.

Care needs to be studied from both humanistic and scientific perspectives, and from the impact of social and cultural forces. It is an issue whether there will be nurses adequately prepared to take this broad and in-depth focus. There are some glimmers of hope (as seen through the yearly National Research Caring and Transcultural Nursing Conferences) that nurses with anthropologic and advanced nursing preparation will provide these perspectives, but we need more nurses involved in and committed to humanistic and scientific care.

Still another issue is how to help nurses value and be committed to care as the essence of nursing—how we can teach and promote care. Even at the International Congress of Nurses held in Los Angeles in 1981, there were no sessions on care except for the presentations by the Transcultural Nursing Society. This transcultural care program had a large number of nurses in attendance, but was ironically not an official part of the program. Several nurses said: "There is hope for the nursing professional with this program, but why is nursing not focusing on care at these international meetings, and especially from a transcultural nursing stance?" Several commented that this care program was the only program focused on care at the International Congress of Nurses. Such comments and others make one realize that nurses are interested in care, but few programs in nursing are focused on the topic.

Still another issue related to care is the teaching of care theories, concepts, and principles to undergraduate and graduate nursing students. The author receives letters and calls daily from nursing students who want to be taught about care or to study care. They are concerned about how few nursing faculty members know about care and teach it. Much of nursing instruction remains focused on medical symptoms, surgical interventions, and technical activities. Students say that they spend far too much time on diseases, body functions, technologic procedures, and drug administration, and very little on care concepts, principles, and research findings. Concepts of presence, support, comfort, and other care measures are only limitedly discussed in most nursing classes. Clinical experiences remain focused on medical activities rather than caring ones. Hence the critical issue remains: How can we prepare faculty and clinical staff to focus on care concepts, processes, and behaviors? Some nursing students seem ahead of their nursing elders in wanting to be taught care and to practice it.

To help students and clinical staff know and practice care further, role models are needed in education and service. We need role models who can teach and demonstrate care components such as support, protection, presence, touch, tenderness, and many others from a biophysiologic, emotional, and cultural viewpoint. Cognitive care models need to promote, demonstrate, and discuss care roles. Comparative role models are needed to prevent cultural imposition on clients of different cultures, and to study different types of care under different conditions or contexts.

Another related issue is the extent to which the nursing profession will support or facilitate incorporation of care concepts or components into the *standards of nursing care*. Currently, such care concepts are not included in nursing care standards. It sounds strange but true, for nursing is an assumed caring profession. To what extent are nurses being certified with thought to their *explicit care knowledge and skills*? To what extent can nurses provide individual and community care that goes *beyond* individual care needs and practices? Such questions and others need discussion.

Still another issue to examine is how to make care an integral part of undergraduate and graduate nursing curricula. What is hindering the inclusion of care in teaching and learning in clinical and home settings? How can faculty be prepared to teach and demonstrate care? Only a few nursing curricula in the country are based on a theory of care.

Another issue is how to encourage the American Nurses Association, National League for Nursing, the American Association of Colleges of Nursing, and other nursing organizations to be active promoters and facilitators of care as part of nursing. Should we introduce a bit of "cultural shock" by highlighting noncare activities of nurses? One can anticipate that nurses will be held legally responsible for noncaring activities and behaviors. We need to have national programs on care with research monies to support its study. National and international papers on care need to be promoted to make care "come alive" to nursing on a national and worldwide basis. What rewards can the national organizations offer for programs focused on care?

There is also the issue of how to help nurses shift to emphasizing care from their past medical services emphasis. Will nursing make this shift? If not, what problems hinder such endeavors? What can be done to help nurses practice care rather than medical assistance activities?

Finally, nurses must encourage the public to remain interested in care as the heart or essence of nursing. The public image of nurses as sophisticated and knowledgeable caregivers could help improve the view of the nursing profession. Public emphasis on care could help differentiate the roles of medicine and nursing in health services. The public seems to want sensitive and knowledgeable care providers, and nurses can be exquisite providers. The author has estimated from interviews with clients that most of them want and expect quality care from health care providers, and less than 20% of clients are really involved in intensive care practices per se.[14] *Care can* and *does* make a difference in recovery from illness and alleviation of actual or potential stresses. Nursing's image could become markedly and positively changed if nurses focused on being exquisite care providers. While there are other issues related to making care a part of the nursing world, the above-mentioned themes are some of the major ones to consider.

In summary, considerable thought, research, and action are needed to make care a *central, unique, dominant,* and *unifying* focus of nursing. *Nursing is caring.* Caring has yet to be explicated and systematically studied as a scientific and humanistic knowledge base of nursing. Many ideas are embedded within the concept of care, such as comfort, support, compassion, presence, and others, yet still too few nurses are studying and committed to care. The comparative care perspective used by transcultural nurses has been invaluable in establishing a growing body of care knowledge. In the future, the author predicts that nursing will make care the major area of study and practice and will conduct the study from a transcultural viewpoint. Nursing students will be explicitly oriented toward knowing and practicing care. Indeed, caring is nursing, and caring is the critical factor that makes a difference in health maintenance and recovery from illness. Caring is culturally based and expressed. When caring is full explicated, and an action is deliberately taken by nurses, then the profession of nursing will at last be publicly recognized. Professional nurses must soon move forward to make caring an integral part of all nursing knowledge and practices, and a fully recognized specialty field. Will nurses take this step and challenge?

REFERENCES

1. Leininger M: Caring: An Essential Human Need. Thorofare, NJ, Charles B. Slack, Inc., 1981.
2. Leininger M: Caring: the essence and central focus of nursing. American Nurses' Foundation (Nursing Research Report) 12(1):2, 14, 1977.
3. Leininger M: The phenomenon of caring: importance, research questions and theoretical considerations. In Leininger M (ed): Caring: An Essential Human Need. Thorofare, NJ, Charles B. Slack, Inc., 1981.
4. Leininger M: Caring: a central focus of nursing and health care services. Nursing and Health Care 1(3):135-143, 176, 1980.
5. Leininger M: Transcultural Nursing: Concepts, Theories and Practices. New York, John Wiley & Sons, 1978.
6. Leininger M: The Gadsup of New Guinea and early child-caring behaviors with nursing care implications. In Leininger M: Transcultural Nursing Concepts, Theories and Practices. New York, John Wiley & Sons, 1978, pp 375-397.
7. Gaut DA: Conceptual analysis of caring: research method. In Leininger M (ed): Caring: An Essential Human Need. Thorofare, NJ, Charles B. Slack, Inc., 1981, pp 18-20.
8. Nightingale F: Notes on Nursing. New York, Dover Publications, 1969.
9. Orem DE: Nursing: concepts of practice. New York, McGraw-Hill Book Company, 1971.
10. Ray M: A study of caring within an institutional culture. Doctoral dissertation, Salt Lake City, University of Utah, August 1981.
11. Leininger M: Towards conceptualization of transcultural health care systems: concepts and a model. In Leininger M: Transcultural Health Care Issues and Conditions. Philadelphia, PA, F.A. Davis Co., 1976.
12. Leininger M: Cross-cultural hypothetical functions of caring and nursing care. In Leininger M (ed): Caring: An Essential Human Need. Thorofare, NJ, Charles B. Slack, Inc., 1981.
13. Leininger M (ed): Proceedings of the National Transcultural Nursing Conferences. New York, Masson International Publishers, 1979.
14. Leininger M: Transcultural Nursing Theories and Research Approaches. In Leininger M: Transcultural Nursing: Concepts, Theories and Practices. New York, John Wiley & Sons, 1978.

8

The Development of a Classification System of Institutional Caring

Professional caring within nursing has been defined largely in relation to an interpersonal process between nurses and clients.[1] From a transcultural nursing perspective, Leininger expanded the notion of caring from an interpersonal process to other levels for research and analytic consideration. In her multilevel structural caring model (individual, family, institutional, cultural, social, and world systems), Leininger proposed that there must be an analysis of the interplay among all levels to gain a more complete knowledge of caring.[1] Thus, to increase caring knowledge within contemporary nursing, it is crucial to the profession to discover its meaning within the specific cultural context of a major social institution—the hospital, wherein many caring activities are carried out.

The purpose of this chapter is to examine the construct of caring as defined by professional nurses and others within the cultural context of the hospital. The ethnonursing research process is outlined. From an in-depth analysis of the caring values and beliefs of the members of the hospital culture, a classification system or a taxonomy is presented, followed by a discussion of the classification system and of the general nature of institutional caring and its relationship to nursing.

THE STUDY OF INSTITUTIONAL CARING

Although "care" and "caring" have been used in nursing literature for more than 100 years, it is only recently that nurses have undertaken systematic philosophic and scientific investigation into the concept. In the past, the author had briefly explored a philosophic approach to caring. She now desires to study caring from an empiric approach utilizing the most familiar of settings—the hospital. An ethnographic study (the descriptive analysis of the cognitions and behaviors of a culture or subculture) was designed to elicit the responses of hospital nurses, clients, and other health and management employees to the primary research question, "How do you define caring, or what does caring mean?" The study had a number of goals and objectives. One of the central objectives was the development of a classification system or a taxonomy of caring which could provide knowledge about the nature of institutional caring. Other goals were established but are not elaborated upon in this chapter.

RESEARCH METHOD

Mishler pointed out that theorists and researchers tend to behave as if context were the enemy of understanding rather than the resource for understanding that it is in our everyday lives.[2] Although the context (or the culture) has been excluded from much of nursing research, especially with respect to experimental design methodology, ethnonursing researchers pursue it as one of the key features in their approach. In this study, context is referred to as "culture," which has been defined by Honigmann as "patterns of learned behaviors and values which are shared among members of a designated group (groups) and usually are transmitted to others of their group (groups) through time."[3] By initiating research within the cultural context of the hospital, we wished to discover the caring values of members of a group or groups of hospital employees, and to develop their caring patterns and trends.

Ethnonursing methodology (the focus on the structure and function of caring integrated within a dynamic culture) dissolves the distinctions between subjects and contexts and according to Wooton explicates the methods by which words are produced and heard as ordered phenomena.[2] By means of the principal method of participant observation, which included the use of the techniques of semistructured or nonstructured interviewing, rigorous documentation, and the use of the analytic tool of comparison, the divergent meanings of caring were determined. Documentation was a crucial analytic process in this ethnonursing field investigation. Mishler characterized the process as a movement through several levels, which represents a movement toward a fuller understanding of the multiple meanings of the (caring) phenomenon—of its coherence, durability, and integrity.[2] Thus, many ethnonursing methods not only were used to collect data, but also were instrumental as investigative tools for understanding the multiplicity of meanings of institutional caring.

The Study Design

The qualitative study was designed in two phases in order to facilitate data collection from participants in the administrative and clinical areas of a religiously-affiliated, urban, acute-care hospital with approximately 350 beds. The data were collected over a total of seven months, with a three-month duration for Phase I (administrative) and a four-month duration for Phase II (clinical). In the clinical phase, participant observation was increased to include the three shift periods. During observations, the researcher went on rounds; attended reports, case conferences, and meetings; sat in on orientation sessions;

and observed day-to-day activities. All interviews were conducted in private, after the "informed consent" documents were signed by the participants. The interviews lasted 35 minutes to two hours. Less formal interviews were also done during the course of the observations.

Sample Selected for The Study

A purposive sample for the administrative phase and a convenience sample for the clinical phase totaling 192 respondents were selected to participate in the caring study. Since this study examined the hospital as a culture and specifically involved nursing, the sample population was not equally represented. Although there is room for biased research in a qualitative study, strong attempts were made to ascertain the validity and reliability of the data by the uses of content, face, and concurrent validity factors and by the repeatability of observations.[4] The technique of frequent comparisons was also used to delineate trends, forms, patterns, and processes of nurses, clients, and administration, as well as their beliefs and practices within the institution.[5,6]

As shown in Table 8-1, nursing participants are represented more than other groups of hospital personnel such as orderlies, housekeepers, and secretaries. A limited number of physicians responded because they were difficult to contact and to engage in nursing research. Also listed in this table is a sample of different cultural group members, especially Hispanics and Blacks. Some important elements of cultural caring were established, but since this subject is not the focal point of this chapter, it is not discussed here.

The ethnonursing research method provided the basis for understanding how members of the hospital community believed and responded to a question about the definition of caring. From the documentation of the qualitative data, an integrated sociology of caring knowledge could be extrapolated. The patterns of institutional caring were complex. One significant pattern discovered through the respondents was the existence of a strong relationship between individual experience and institutional functioning.

RESULTS: THE DEVELOPMENT OF AN INSTITUTIONAL CARING CLASSIFICATION SYSTEM

An analysis of the cognitions of the participants in this study provided the foundation from which a classification (taxonomy or naming) system could be developed. Leininger summarized the general features of a taxonomy as: (1) an orderly way to arrange and study data at an early or final stage; (2) a conceptual structure to determine what is included or excluded on the subject; (3) a ranking of large and small units of a phenomenon with subcategories according to knowledge about each domain; and (4) a dynamic or change structure used to accommodate new knowledge about the phenomenon under study.[1]

Table 8-2 is a presentation of the respondents' categories of caring, listing the total number of responses to the research question regarding the definition of caring. They were categorized (psychologic, practical, interactive, and philosophic) by the researcher in the process of data analysis. "Categories" are defined by Spradley as primary types of cultural symbols (verbal and nonverbal), or symbols that assist in the decoding of meaning.[7] In Table 8-2, the four major cognitive categories, listed in decreasing order by the number of responses, are kinds of verbal cultural caring symbols. These caring symbols were interpreted, and their meaning was derived logically by the researcher.

In Table 8-3, caring responses of different nurse groups according to their educational preparation are presented. The findings revealed that there was little difference in the average number of total caring responses between nurse-administrators and registered staff nurses. However, the licensed practical nurse/technician group had a slightly higher response average than registered nurses. Most of the nurses had diploma education, but 39% also had advanced educational preparation—Bachelor of Science or Master of Arts or Science degrees.

Table 8-4 shows the caring classification system. The verbal cultural caring symbols (Level 1) with their subcategories (Levels 2 and 3) are defined as the following:

1. *Psychologic.* (a) *Affective*—relating to, arising from, or influencing feelings or emotions, expressing emotion, eg, love; (b) *Cognitive*—relating to knowledge used to define and interpret actions and events, eg, decision.

2. *Practical.* (a) *Social Organization*—relating to the practical consideration and activities of the sociocultural environment, eg, political, legal, economic, and social structural characteristics; (b) *Technical*—relating to techniques, principles, and/or methods, or use of technology to achieve a therapeutic purpose, eg, skill.

3. *Interactional.* (a) *Physical*—relating to the body, nonverbal communication for the purpose of providing physical comfort, eg, touch; (b) *Social*—relating to interpersonal reciprocal action for the purpose of therapeutic outcomes, eg, communication.

4. *Philosophic.* (a) *Spiritual*—relating to matters of a sacred nature, eg, prayer, virtuous or ritual acts, acts of faith, relation of man/woman with God; (b) *Ethical*—relating to implications of morality, right or wrong, professional or organizational principles of honor or virtue, eg, trust; (c) *Culture*—relating to perceptions, attitude, and knowledge of the caring needs of persons of different cultural/ethnic groups within the hospital.

Text continues on p. 103.

Table 8-1. Demographic Features of Role Participants

Group	Role	Number			Culture Groups (other than white)				
		Males	Females	Total	Hispanic	Black	Oriental	Other	Total
Administrator	Nonnurse	11	17	28		1			1
	Nurse	2	35	37	3	1	1		5
Staff	RN	3	47	50	3	1	1	1	6
	Technicians/ LPN	1	15	16		4			4
	Aide		9	9	2	2			4
	Orderly	2		2					
	Guard	1		1					
	Housekeeper	1	2	3	1	1			2
	Secretary		1	1					
Other	Physician	5	1	6					
	Student	1	11	12					
	Client	15	11	26	4	3		5	11
	Educator		1	1					
Total	14	42	150	192	13	13	2	5	33

Table 8-2. Cognitive Caring Categories of Hospital Participants

Role	No.	Psychological	Practical	Interactive	Philosophic	No. of Caring Responses
Nonnurse Administrators	28	68	78	50	44	240
Nurse-Adm.	37	87	111	63	67	328
RN-Staff Nurse	50	145	107	98	84	434
LPN/Technician	16	24	25	34	13	96
Aides	9	17	9	14	9	49
Orderly	2	4	3	1	3	11
Guards	1		1	1		2
Housekeepers	3		3	1	1	5
Secretary	1	1	1	2	2	6
Physicians	6	7	14	4	1	26
Students (BS)	12	25	5	10	6	46
Clients	26	43	2	37	26	108
Educators	1	1	3	3	1	11
Total	192	425	362	318	257	1362

Table 8-3. Nurses' Roles, Educational Preparation, and Years and Types of Nursing Experience

Role	Number			Educational Preparation[a]			Years of Experience				Types of Experience			
	Respondents	Caring Responses	% Average	Diploma	BS	MA/MS	Less than 10	10-20	21-30	31-40	H[b]	PH[c]	NH[d]	ED[e]
RN Administrator	37	328	10.3	26	13	5	10	18	3	6	37	2		
RN Staff	50	434	11.5	40	14	2	28	10	5	7	50	1	1	2
LPN/Technician	16	96	16	16			14	2			16		4	
Total	103	858		82	27	7	52	30	8	13	103	3	5	2

[a]Some respondents have more than one type of education.

[b]Hospital, [c]Public Health, [d]Nursing Home, [e]Education

Table 8-4. Classification of Cognitive Perceptions of Caring

Level 1[b]	Cognitive Categories Level 2	Level 3	Caring Characteristics[a] Expressions
Psychologic	A. Affective	A. Feeling	A. Empathy
	B. Cognitive	B. Knowing	B. Meeting Needs
Practical	A. Social Organization	A. Indirect/ Direct	A. Economic/ Budget/Money
	B. Technical	B. Indirect/ Direct	B. Skill
Inter- actional	A. Physical	A. Doing for	A. Touch
	B. Social	B. Doing with	B. Communica- tion/Talking
Philo- sophic	A. Spiritual	A. Moral Concern	A. Spiritual Needs
	B. Ethical	B. Moral Concern	B. Attitude
	C. Cultural	C. Concern	C. Equity

[a]Example only. See Tables 8–5—8–8 for complete range of characteristics.

[b]Level 1 ranked highest to lowest in terms of caring responses.

These categories are the bridge between the practical definitions of the participants and the abstract thinking of the investigator.

Durkheim and Mauss claimed that in a classification system, related ideas can be grouped and arranged hierarchically.[8] Also, Spradley stated that a taxonomy is the internal structure of a unit of cultural knowledge, which always approximates the way in which respondents have arranged that knowledge.[7] This study of caring supports those claims through its groups and hierarchic arrangements. Moreover, Levels 2 and 3 represent a further refinement of the meaning of caring; Level 2 refers to the types of meaning, and Level 3 refers to the functions or the functional relationships that are associated with the meanings of each category.

Table 8-5 shows the characteristics of caring in the psychologic category—the first in the hierarchic ordering of caring because it has the greatest number of responses. Those characteristics concerned with the knowledge level of the psychologic category were rated the highest, indicating that professionally, factors relating to "knowing" are necessary and important to providing care to clients within the institution. This notion is supported by Mayeroff, who stated the following: "To care for someone, I must *know* many things. I must know, for example, who the other is, what his power and limitations are, and what is conducive to his (her) growth; I must know how to respond to his (her) needs, and what my own powers and limitations are. Such knowledge is both general and specific."[9]

Table 8-5 also shows the affective or "feeling" characteristics of psychologic caring. Respondents generally presented these ideas at the outset of the interview, thus pointing to the primary importance of the humanistic or "ideal" dimension of caring. Although the more humanistic dimensions of caring were preferred, nurses' affective definitions only slightly outnumbered statements referring to their roles and statements that caring is bound to the functioning of the organization.

In Table 8-6, definitions of caring and its relationship to the organization were identified, ranking the practical category second within the hierarchic structure of caring. The social organizational level was linked largely to the economy, and to the coordination of activities and time. Under the technical level, skill (both physical and technologic) was the top response. Caring was connected strongly with practical issues; this represented its changing posture within the context of the hospital.[5]

Table 8-7 represents the interactional category, and is the third of the four categories in the caring structure. The social aspects of interaction outranked physical interaction, and the table shows that communication (talking) incurred the greatest number of responses. Bell predicted that information would be the major criterion in postindustrial society.[10] Thus, in the organizational system of the hospital, information in the form of communication-interaction must be one of the crucial areas of bureaucratic management and concentration.

Text continues on p. 107.

Table 8-5. Characteristics of Caring—Psychologic Category

Categories			Characteristics	No. of Responses
Level 1	Level 2	Level 3		
Psychologic	A. Affective	A. Feeling	Empathy	33
			Concern	31
			Feeling	22
			Loving	18
			Compassion	14
			Givingness	12
			Friendliness (Closeness)	10
			Enjoyment	9
			Sympathy (Understanding)	9
			Patience	8
			Sensitivity	8
			Kindness	7
			Interest	6
			Motivation	4
			Cheerfulness	3
			Intimacy	2
			Strength	2
			Tenderness	2
			Peak Experience	1
			Vulnerability	1
			N =	202
	B. Cognitive	B. Knowing	Teaching	52
			Meeting Needs	40
			Knowledge	33
			Observation (Watchover)	28
			Decisions	21
			Assessment	18
			Evaluation	15
			Problem Solving	11
			Integration	4
			Intuition	1
			N =	223
			TOTAL =	425

Table 8-6. Characteristics of Caring—Practical Category

Categories			Characteristics	No. of Responses
Level 1	Level 2	Level 3		
Practical	A. Social Organization	A. Indirect/ Direct	Economic/Money Budget	61
			Organization/ Coordination	41
			Time	36
			Legal/Defensive	26
			Presence (Being There/ Availability)	21
			Political Competition	20
			Safety	20
			Paperwork/ Charting	20
			Woman's Movement	10
			Control	7
			Policy-Making	5
			Audit	3
			Provision of activities	1
			Managerial Development	1
			N =	272
	B. Technical	B. Indirect/ Direct	Skill	71
			Equipment Maintenance/ Design	14
			Technologic/ Diagnostic Research	3
			Scientific Care	1
			Therapeutic Maintenance	1
			N =	90
			TOTAL =	362

Table 8-7. Characteristics of Caring—Interactional Category

Categories			Characteristics	No. of Responses
Level 1	**Level 2**	**Level 3**		
Interactional	A. Physical	A. Doing for	Comfort (Physical)	41
			Touch	36
			N =	77
	B. Social	B. Doing with	Communication (Talking)	80
			Interact (Share)	44
			Listen	32
			Help	27
			Involve	14
			Reassure	13
			Support	11
			Counsel	8
			Rapport	6
			Protect	4
			Nurture	2
			N =	241
			TOTAL =	318

Table 8-8 represents the final category of the organizational caring structure, receiving the least number of responses. The philosophic category consisted of three levels of meaning—spiritual, ethical, and cultural.

Many clients, especially those who were near death, emphasized spiritual concerns, and stated how much the meaning of caring was a part of their response to suffering, a response that they ultimately linked to faith in God. Personnel from religious orders, middle-aged nursing staff, and other long-term employees referred to spirituality as a definition of caring, but emphasized how the institution had changed. For example, spirituality now was "categorized" into a department (Pastoral Care) rather than being an integral part of each individual's responsibility in the organization.

The ethical level produced the greatest number of caring responses in the philosophic category. Several respondents stated that "attitude" was a factor in caring, and several expressed concern about the shift from "other-oriented" service to more "self-centered" interests.

A separate category for cultural characteristics of the participants was not developed. Cultural responses were placed in Table 8-8 under the philosophic category because from a professional standpoint, the term "cultural care" continues to be more philosophic than an integral part of interactive care.

DISCUSSION: THE MEANING OF INSTITUTIONAL CARING

Interpreting the meaning of thought and conduct within a culture is the central aim of ethnonursing. "Meaning, in one form or another, permeates the experience of most human beings in all societies," claimed Spradley.[5] Moreover, Mishler pointed out that "meaning is always within context and context incorporates meaning. Both are produced by human actors through their actions."[2] Consequently, in analyzing and categorizing knowledge about caring, the linguistic elements of communicating meaning are critical components.

In a study of institutional caring, the cognitive definitions (although artificially categorized for the purposes of research) demonstrated their integral relationship to the social and cultural environment. This interconnectedness between individuals and their environment has been labeled in anthropology as the field of culture and personality. LeVine claimed, "Nothing is more characteristic of the field of culture and personality than its concern with the transactions between the microsocial domain of individual experience and the macrosocial domain of institutional functioning."[11] This interconnectedness can increase our understanding of the impact of social institutions on behavior.

In examining the response rates of caring definitions across the categories, the psychologic category ranked the highest in terms of caring responses (at 425), followed by the practical category, with 362 responses. The interactive and philosophic categories ranked third and fourth, with 318 and 257 responses,

Table 8-8. Characteristics of Caring—Philosophic Category

Categories			Characteristics	No. of Responses
Level 1	Level 2	Level 3		
Philosophic	A. Spiritual	A. Moral Concern	Spiritual Concern	18
			Faith	8
			Healing	1
			Christian Philosophy (Doing for Others)	1
			Authenticity	1
			Belongingness	1
			N =	30
	B. Ethical	B. Moral Concern	Attitude	27
			Responsibility	24
			Holistic Care	23
			Trust	20
			Individualistic Care	20
			Respect	20
			Self-Care	9
			Humanness	7
			Dedication	6
			Ethics/Truth	6
			Commitment	3
			Patient Advocate	3
			Honesty	2
			Sincerity	2
			Loyalty	1
			N =	173
	C. Cultural	C. Concern	Some understanding of cultural care (interpretors)	30
			Equity in Cultural Care	14
			No. of understanding cultural care	6
			Class Care	4
			N =	54
			TOTAL =	257

respectively. Universal definitions or meanings of caring in nursing, and other disciplines such as philosophy and psychology, generally refer to caring as having affective or humanistic characteristics. Thus, the fact that the psychologic category ranked the highest was not surprising. The interactive category ranked third in the hierarchic caring structure, which could also be anticipated by the researcher, especially given the emphases on verbal and nonverbal educational socialization practices in the past decade among health personnel. However, what was not anticipated was the shift in the interpretation of caring from its traditional religious-philosophic dimensions to more political and economic ones, as noted in the hierarchic structural position of both the practical and philosophic categories. Respondents emphatically remarked that hospital caring was now a "big business," and financial administrators often referred to caring as a function of the hospital's economic health.[12]

Changes in the structural caring elements of the hospital social organization are influenced by changes in the dominant culture. Bevis documented that historically, nursing's values and behavior reflected society's values and attitudes. She identified four philosophic trends in the history of nursing, the most recent trend being "humanism."[13] Ethnonursing data from this study suggested that humanistic dimensions have been enlarged to include the influences of the organizational social structural elements. Although the "humanistic" dimensions of caring were declared by nurses and others to be the highest-ranking category, participant-observation research strategies revealed that the technologic, political, economic, and legal systems were dominating the hospital caring culture. This shift toward the incorporation of more practical considerations into the meaning of caring must be a serious query for all members of the institutional community. What is the extent of the relationship between bureaucracy and caring?

The research data from this study of caring suggested a qualitatively strong relationship. How has nursing been affected? Direct interpersonal client-care interaction wherein humanistic caring could be practiced was not seen as the most fulfilling or rewarding role. Many nurses reported that they were interested in leaving nursing to find other jobs with better benefits and less responsibility. In support of this, documentation of recruitment and retention facts published by the National League for Nursing shows a decline in persons entering and remaining in nursing.[14] The humanistic value system of nursing now is being challenged by nurses themselves. Nurses in this study no longer saw themselves as completely dedicated to the causes of clients, physicians, and the hospital. As one nurse with 36 years of experience claimed, "You can't live on dedication!" Another nurse reported that "the important things in nursing right now are woman's liberation, low pay, and 'burn-out.' "

By attempting to seek more advancement, recognition, and economic gain within or outside the hospital, conflicts and contradictions have emerged among the caring ideologies of nurses, the institution, and the dominant cultural system. What is the deeper meaning behind these conflicts? A simple explanation could be placing blame on one group or another or on society, and claiming that no one cares anymore. People do care, however. What is different are *the types of caring*. For the administration, economic and political concerns were interpreted as caring. Accordingly, the effective management of money, time, and people were important to the functioning of the hospital. For many of the staff nursing personnel, there was a dramatic change from the traditional "otherness" orientation to "self" reflection. Nurses' unmet needs, that is, the lack of personal reward in providing care, the failure of open communication, and the deficiencies of the nurses' economic system, resulted in overt and covert threats of union development, and most alarmingly, the burn-out syndrome. These factors led many to feelings of alienation, depression, and hopelessness, and to desertion of their professional commitments or careers, or both.

The psychologic, practical, interactive, and philosophic caring categories developed in this study highlighted the notion of interconnectedness between individuals and their environment. When evaluating the numeric responses of participants, the combined psychologic, interactive, and philosophic categories dominated the cognitive structure of institutional caring. In contrast, however, the practical category *strongly* influenced the nature of most of the interviews about caring. Consequently, in many ways, the political, legal, and economic systems of the bureaucracy, although not negative in themselves, dwarfed the more universal, positive elements of ethico-spiritual-humanistic caring. A new kind of "social linkage" to caring now is necessary, especially for nurses. Animosities created by altered ideologies, institutional exploitation, and interprofessional competition must be transformed so as to lead to a more politically equitable bureaucratic environment. There is a need for action to stimulate and heighten commitment, intent, and purpose. The author believes that caring within an institutional framework clearly rests on an increasing knowledge of the social structural elements (political, legal, technologic, social, and economic, in conjunction with the ethico-spiritual-humanistic elements). "Bureaucratization" is gaining greater prominence in social development.[10] Britan and Cohen cogently state the following:

> Like it or not, humankind is being driven to a bureaucratized world whose forms and functions, whose authority and power, must be understood if they are ever to be even partially controlled.[15]

Given the dynamic process of increasing bureaucracy in world culture, bureaucracy and nursing require immediate attention. The future of nursing within the institution depends on how well the synthetic nature of bureaucratic caring in a positive and growth-producing sense is understood. What are the beneficial components of bureaucracy; ie, what are the political, economic, social, and technologic caring factors, and what are their epiphenomena (another side of the same coin) that are capable of destroying the profession? As world society grows in complexity, the consciousness of nursing and institutional caring must also grow.

SUMMARY

The development of a classification system and the analysis of institutional caring structures represented by Tables 8-1 to 8-8 were the point of discussion of this chapter. Durkheim and Mauss stated that the object of a classification system was to advance understanding by making intelligible how each category stands in relation to another category, and how together they form the whole.[8] The classification of caring in an institutional context advanced our understanding of its complex nature, as well as illustrated its logical structure of distinct yet interrelated categories: psychologic, practical, interactional, and philosophic.

Durkheim and Mauss further pointed to the fact that a "logical hierarchy is only another aspect of the social hierarchy, and the unity of knowledge is nothing else than the very unit of the collectivity, extended to the universe."[8]

Similarly, the categories of caring evolved from specific definitions of the concept showed that the relationships among the individual, the social organization, and the society provided a basis for the structural unity of caring knowledge. Despite the discovery of the structural unity of institutional caring knowledge, however, it has not promoted, as yet, a spirit of optimism, hope, or a vehicle for personal growth for the nursing profession within the hospital culture. Nursing's future as a profession is dependent not only upon the expansion of its humanistic caring dimensions, but also upon the development of its pragmatic (social structural) dimensions. Bevis wrote that "humanistic existentialism seems to be the natural maturational philosophy for nursing."[11,13] However, this study pointed to the fact that the primary humanistic dimension of caring has rapidly expanded to include other social structural characteristics. The tension that exists between the ideal elements of humanism and the material structure of bureaucracy offers the greatest challenge to nursing. Given this task, nurses and others will be called to discover the ideal in the real world, and to work toward the construction of deeper levels of meaning of caring knowledge within contemporary institutional cultures.

REFERENCES

1. Leininger M (ed): Caring: An Essential Human Need. Proceedings of the Three National Caring Conferences. Thorofare, NJ, Charles B. Slack, Inc., 1981.
2. Mishler EG: Meaning in context. Is there any other kind? Harvard Educational Review 49(2):1-19, 1979.
3. Leininger M: Transcultural Nursing: Concepts, Theories and Practices. New York, John Wiley & Sons, 1978, p 60.
4. Geertz C: The Interpretation of Cultures. New York, Basic Books, Inc., 1973.
5. Leininger M: Ethnonursing research methods (Class notes). Salt Lake City, University of Utah, 1977, 1978.
6. Glaser B, Strauss A: The Discovery of Grounded Theory: Strategies for Qualitative Research. Chicago, Aldine Publishing Co., 1967.
7. Spradley JP: The Ethnographic Interview. New York, Holt, Rinehart and Winston, 1979.
8. Durkheim E, Mauss M: Primitive Classification. Needham R(trans.). Chicago, IL, The University of Chicago Press, Phoenix Books, 1967.
9. Mayeroff M: On Caring. New York, Harper and Row, 1971, p 9.

10. Bell D: The Coming of Post-Industrial Society. New York, Basic Books Inc., 1974.
11. LeVine R: Culture, Behavior and Personality. Chicago, Aldine Publishing Co., 1973, p 12.
12. Perrow C: Complex Organizations: A Critical Essay, 2nd ed. Glenview, IL, Scott, Foresman and Co., 1979.
13. Bevis EO: Curriculum Building in Nursing, 2nd ed. St. Louis, MO, C.V. Mosby Co., 1978.
14. National League for Nursing (NLN): Facts about nursing. New York, April, 1981.
15. Britan GM, Cohen R (eds): Hierarchy and Society. Philadelphia, PA, ASHI, 1980, p 27.

9

Self-Care and Caretaking of The Adolescent Asthmatic Girl

The purpose of this chapter is to gather information according to the protocol of the ethnographic interview and to develop ethnographic statements and culturally relevant descriptions concerning an aspect of the life of the adolescent asthmatic girl.[1] The specific aspect to be considered is how adolescent girls with moderate to severe asthma view their relationships with their age mates. The research question addressed in the study is: "What knowledge do adolescent asthmatic girls use to generate behavior and interpret experience during interaction with their peers?"[2]

The systematic use of the ethnographic interview enabled the researcher to gather precise detail and description regarding the culture of the adolescent asthmatic girl. One of the tasks of the ethnographic interview is to discover domains or categories of information for organizing human experience. The prevailing theme discovered throughout the data collection focused on care— how the adolescent asthmatic girl cares for herself, and how she perceives herself as a recipient of care.

This chapter describes the research performed and display data collected and, finally, suggests caring components and constructs.

The culture chosen for study included adolescent girls with moderate to severe asthma. In order to study the selected culture within a relevant framework, the girls were interviewed regarding their perceptions of peer relationships.

The adolescent asthmatic children involved in the study were between the ages of 11 and 16 years. Chronic illness, including asthma, is seen as a major challenge to nursing, medicine, and families with chronic illness. The challenge is increased with the severity of the disease and the length of time the adolescent has been chronically ill with asthma.[3]

During adolescence, there is nothing more important to the child than peer relationships.[4] The concept of peer group is drawn from the work of Ausubel,

Montemayor, and Svajian.[4] These authors spoke of the emotional support the peer group offers and the selectivity involved. The emotional support derived from the peer group provides a springboard from which the adolescent is able to make great strides toward emancipation from parents, home, and childhood. Greater selectivity in the organization and composition of peer groups is the discriminating factor between childhood peer groups and those of adolescence.

Using the concept of peer group, Ausubel et al identified three categories of socially rejected adolescents.[4] They are as follows:

1. Individuals who are rejected by the group because of personality traits, physical characteristics, or interests.

2. Individuals who reject the group because they find the association unrewarding or traumatic.

3. Those who neither reject nor are rejected, but accept ostracism in order to pursue other needs and interests.[4]

Chronic illness may result in personality traits or physical characteristics that are unacceptable to the peer group. Adolescents with chronic illness can be candidates for the first category of socially rejected adolescents.

CONCEPTUAL FRAMEWORK

The concepts of adolescence, peer groups, chronic illness (the asthma experience), and the ethnographic interview are the basis of this research and compose the conceptual framework. Statements that summarize the conceptual framework are:

- Adolescents, experiencing a period of rapid and progressive change, depend on their peer group for emotional support.

- Peer groups are characterized by selectivity and intolerance of imperfection.

- The asthma experience of chronic illness affects all aspects of the adolescent's life, including peer relations.

- The ethnographic interview is a systematic method of studying adolescent asthmatic girls from the point of view of a member of their culture, in order to construct a model of a cultural system that guides their behavior during peer relationships.

METHOD

Ethnoscientists view cultures as systems of knowledge. This view supports the theory of cultures as ideologic systems as opposed to cultures as adaptive and dynamic systems.[5] Spradley has pursued the use of the ethnographic method in queries of behavioral determinants.[1]

The nature of culture can be better appreciated and understood via field work. Field work is necessary to gain a high level of concept comprehension.[5] Cultural deliberation must also recognize that "variations among individuals of similar cultural heritage enlarge the complexity of providing quality health care in transcultural settings."[6]

Leininger unites transcultural considerations and nursing theory with the statement: "Transcultural nursing theory refers to a set of interrelated cross-cultural nursing concepts and hypotheses which take into account individual and group caring behaviors, values, beliefs based upon their cultural needs, in order to provide effective and satisfying nursing care to people; and if such nursing practices fail to recognize culturological aspects of human needs, there will be signs of less efficacious nursing care practices and some unfavorable consequences to those served."[6]

As mentioned previously, for the purpose of the study, the ethnographic interview was useful because this method provided a systematic approach for getting to the native's cultural viewpoint. The information that the members of a culture possess is highly organized and fits together in a meaningful way. The basic premise of this method is that information is gathered directly from informants. The collected information gives clues to the cognitive map or knowledge of the informant's culture. Initially, the ethnographic interview resembles a friendly conversation. The researcher slowly introduces new questions to assist the informants to act as information sharers. The researcher often begins with a "grand tour," or descriptive type of question to encourage the informant to provide a verbal picture of a particular cultural scene.[1] Some of the "grand tour" questions used in this research were, "What kinds of things happen during a typical school day?", "What kinds of things do you and your friends do for fun?", and "What kinds of things do you do for your friends and do your friends do for you?" Answers provided by the informants are used to discover other culturally relevant questions.

During the research, data were collected from four adolescent asthmatic girls, ranging in age from 11 to 16 years. All were English speaking, had had severe asthma since preschool, had been hospitalized for their asthma since that time, took medications routinely for their asthma, and were willing to participate in the study. Girls were chosen as subjects, since the researcher is also a woman, and it was felt that the research would be facilitated by studying subjects of the same sex. Each girl was interviewed four times: the interviews were approximately 45 minutes to one hour in duration. The interviews were taped and the settings were private, with only the informant and researcher present. Throughout the interview, data were collected which would lead to the discovery of cultural themes.

Cultural themes give clues for tying together bits and pieces of data collected from members of a culture. They expose the elements of a complex pattern. The themes present a holistic view of a culture in recurrent strands which run through two or more domains. The cultural themes discovered during the research were, "Friends are sensitive and understanding," "Control your asthma or it will control you," "Asthmatics are different," and "Asthma isn't everything." These themes are discussed briefly, and then examples of the data follow.

"Friends are sensitive and understanding" includes the categories of sensitive yet normal treatment for an asthmatic, and personal yet technical understanding of the disease process. Understanding involves two primary components: technical knowledge of asthma as a disease, and personal knowledge of the adolescent with asthma. These two components provide an organizing frame of reference for experiences with an asthmatic friend during an asthma crisis.

The second cultural theme is "control your asthma or it will control you." The concept of "control" refers to a continuous power struggle with physical, emotional, and environmental factors influencing the client's power struggle.[7]

"Asthmatics are different," the third cultural theme, demonstrates that the informants viewed themselves as being different from their nonasthmatic peers. The informants cited examples of emotional and physical constraints.

The final theme, "asthma isn't everything," does not negate the effect of asthma on all facets of life. Asthma is important but not the beginning and end of the asthmatic girls' existence. Despite their chronic conditions, the informants view themselves as functioning at satisfactory levels. The informants have developed their strengths, including intellectual, musical, and athletic abilities. Disabilities are accepted and minimized. One of the informants was asked if she thought she would be any different if she did not have asthma, to which she replied, "No, I think I would be about the same."

ASTHMA AND SELF-CARE

Hyde states: "Caring for ourselves and others is based on the self care of liking, valuing and accepting ourselves. In harmony with our own core of deepest values, we reach out to care for others in our world."[8] She further identifies the key issues of self-care and caring as motivation and decision.

The category "asthma and self-care" was described by at least one of the children. The data collected demonstrate schematically how adolescent asthmatic girls organize their knowledge of how they take care of themselves (see Table 9–1).

This form of information display is called a "taxonomy." In the complete taxonomy entitled "Things She Does for Her Asthma," there are four major categories arranged to the left, and then each is broken down into more detail. In Table 9–1, included in the category "things that are good for her" are as follows: eat right, exercise, watch the weather, get allergy shots, keep the house clean, see the doctor, and don't overdo it. "Don't overdo it" is further divided into don't run, don't walk too far, don't go to bed too late, and don't get overweight. Other self-care activities include things she has to do, things that mean she's an addict, and things she does that make her different. All the data have been recorded in the same words the children used.

Table 9-1. Asthma and Self-Care

	EAT RIGHT	{ WATCH CALORIES WATCH ALLERGIES
	EXERCISE	
	WATCH THE WEATHER	
THINGS THAT ARE GOOD FOR HER	GET ALLERGY SHOTS	
	KEEP THE HOUSE CLEAN	
	SEE THE DOCTOR	
	DON'T OVERDO IT	{ DON'T RUN DON'T WALK TOO FAR DON'T GO TO BED TOO LATE DON'T GET OVERWEIGHT

CARETAKING OF THE ASTHMATIC

The children were able to break down the category of things friends do for them into three parts, consisting of those behaviors that the adolescent asthmatic identifies as bad, maybe, or good. Whether the behavior is categorized as bad, maybe, or good depends on the doer's intent and the circumstances (Table 9-2). Not all the behaviors are necessarily related to asthma, but some address problems the adolescent faces on a day-to-day basis.

Table 9-2. Caretaking Activities of Friends

BAD	TREAT HER LIKE A BABY PROTECT HER GET WATER FOR HER FEEL SORRY FOR HER, BUT DON'T TELL HER BRING ATTENTION TO HER ASTHMA
MAYBE	TAKE CARE OF HER CALM HER DOWN A LITTLE DON'T IGNORE HER (HAVING AN ATTACK) ASSIGN JOBS SHE CAN DO
GOOD	MIND THEIR MANNERS DO FAVORS FOR HER STAY CLOSE WHEN WHEEZING UNDERSTAND HER MOVE TO ARIZONA

THE ASTHMA CRISIS

The description of the asthma crisis gave rise to a taxonomy, a paradigm, and a flow chart. The taxonomy "Things That Happen During an Asthma Attack" includes the things the child feels, the things others do, and medications taken (Table 9-3). Things that others do include things Mom does, things Dad does, and things other visitors in the home do.

Table 9-3. Things That Happen During An Asthma Attack

	FEEL THINGS	CRAMP IN SIDES OF CHEST
		LITTLE THING GOES IN AND OUT
		COUGH
		SHORTNESS OF BREATH
		WHEEZE
		REALLY BAD STING
THINGS THAT HAPPEN AT HOME	OTHERS DO	MOM DOES
		DAD DOES
		VISITORS DO
	TAKE MEDICINE	METAPREL
		MIST
		SHOT

The paradigm presents data in another fashion. The paradigm utilizes dimensions required to discriminate between pieces of cultural data. The paradigm shown in Table 9-4 indicates how the child differentiates among the events that occur during an asthma crisis. The flow chart, Figure 9-1, reveals another method of data display and depicts how the information concerning an asthma crisis was organized in the mind of one of the informants.

Figure 9-1 demonstrates the primary theme of "WAIT," and this term is shown to connect the events. "Waiting" poignantly represents the lack of control that each child felt during the crisis.

If the x-ray indicates that there is an infection in the child's lungs, then the child must WAIT to be admitted. The children felt that with appropriate intervention (not always external), the attack could dissipate and the child would return to status quo. If control is not regained, the attack progresses, very probably to hospitalization.

Table 9-4. Componential Definitions of Contrast in Things That Happen During An Asthma Attack

N=NO
Y=YES
S=SOMETIMES
NA=NOT APPLICABLE

	MOM KNOWS	IT WORKS/HELPS/ FEELS BETTER	DO IT AGAIN	HAPPENS AT NIGHT	NOTICE IT HAPPENS	REALLY IMPORTANT
USE METAPREL	S	S	Y	Y	Y	Y
DAD GIVES SHOT	Y	S	N	Y	Y	Y
NICE NURSE GIVES HER STUFF SHE NEEDS	N	Y	N	Y	Y	N

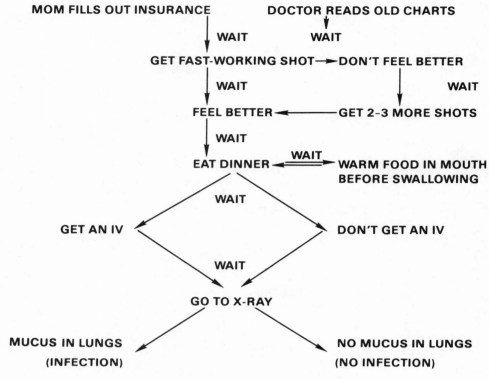

Figure 9–1. Flowchart of an asthma crisis.

CARING COMPONENTS AND CONSTRUCTS

The ethnographic method does not recognize the privilege of interpretation. However, in a perusal of Leininger's 30 Major Taxonomic Caring Constructs, six of those constructs are glaringly evident in the data collected. These constructs include interest, health maintenance acts, presence, protective behaviors, sharing, and surveillance.[6,9] Five other caring components are also evident in the review of the data, such as sensitivity, valuing, understanding, acceptance, and liking. Differentiation among these components has not been studied by this researcher. Therefore, some of the components and constructs are combined in specific examples.

Sensitivity and understanding have already been described in the first cultural theme, "friends are sensitive and understanding." The component identified as understanding refers to technical knowledge of asthma and personal knowledge of the adolescent with asthma.

Protective behaviors included those acts that serve as guards against episodes of sensitivity. An example is the child who is intensely sensitive to peanut butter.

Protective behaviors specifically are "not blowing peanut butter breath in her face" and "not leaving a peanut butter knife in the sink when she has to do the dishes."

Interest and sharing are tremendously important to adolescents in general, who are struggling through rapid and progressive changes over which they have little control.

Presence and surveillance are not well differentiated. An example is when the child is wheezing and possibly experiencing some difficulty in breathing. At this point, friends will demonstrate their presence through proximity, and their surveillance through a readiness to react hastily should their asthmatic friend require such care.

Health maintenance acts were performed via self-care behaviors such as "eat right" and "keep the house clean." Acts demonstrated by those around the adolescent asthmatic girl are Mom, who "calls the doctor," and Dad, who "gives the shot."

It would be virtually impossible for an adolescent asthmatic girl to perform self-care if she did not value, accept, and like herself. Noncompliance during certain periods in her life indicate that these components may be dynamic and variable.

CONCLUSIONS

Communication of cultural knowledge is a skill that the professional nurse is expected to perfect.[10] Communication is encouraged among health professionals, but the researcher suggests the dissemination of knowledge of human behavior and development beyond the confines of nursing and medicine. It is recommended that knowledge of adolescent asthmatics acquired in practice and research be shared with other individuals working and involved with adolescent asthmatics, such as educators and parents. Methods for the dissemination of knowledge include publication, further research, and interdisciplinary exchanges.

Recommendations for further research in this area include replication of the study with fewer or more informants and interviewing more than four times; replication of the study using a group setting rather than the individual approach; replication with informants of different age, sex, and degree of illness; and replication with different chronic diseases.

It is the responsibility of nurse researchers to use ethnographic research to generate questions that lend themselves to further research. The following questions are submitted:

1. Do asthmatics view themselves differently at different ages?

2. Could a taxonomy of a culturally relevant domain lend itself to the formation of a nursing assessment tool for the adolescent asthmatic girl?

3. What information do children want nurses to know and are therefore willing to impart to the nurse?

4. Will the study of the self-care and caretaking behaviors of the adolescent contribute to the understanding of nursing as a caring profession?

REFERENCES

1. Spradley J: The Ethnographic Interview. New York, Holt, Rinehart and Winston, 1979.
2. Mennen MS: The world of the adolescent asthmatic girl. Unpublished master's thesis, University of Arizona, Tucson, AZ, 1970.
3. Kugelmass I: Adolescent Medicine: Principles and Practice. Springfield, IL, Charles C Thomas, 1975.
4. Ausubel D, Montemayor R, Svajian P: Theory and Problems of Adolescent Development. New York, Grune and Stratton, 1977.
5. Spradley J, McCurdy D: The Cultural Experience Ethnography in Complex Society. Chicago, Science Research Associates, Inc., 1972.
6. Leininger M: Transcultural Nursing: Concepts, Theories and Practices. New York, John Wiley and Sons, 1978, p 33.
7. Bergner M, Hutelmyer C: Teaching kids how to live with their allergies. Nursing 6(8):11, 1976.
8. Hyde A: The phenomenon of caring. American Nurses' Foundation (Nursing Research Report) 11(1):2, 1976.
9. Leininger M: The phenomenon of caring: importance, research questions and theoretical considerations. *In* Leininger M (ed): Caring: An Essential Human Need. Proceedings of the Three National Caring Conferences. Thorofare, NJ, Charles B. Slack, Inc., 1981, pp 133–143.
10. Aamodt A: Culture. *In* Culture Childbearing Health Professionals. Philadelphia, PA, F.A. Davis Co., 1979.

10

Indigenous Caring Practices In a Guatemalan Colonia

Many developing countries, including those in Latin America, are not giving priority to providing primary health care to underserved populations. The expansion of preventive-oriented services underscores how important it is for nurses to have a basis for meeting health needs within different cultural and international settings. Increasingly, within each country, nurses are assuming responsibility for designing and implementing health care programs. The basis for understanding and planning primary health care services within each cultural context is an understanding of how clients experience situations and events that influence the maintenance and promotion of health. Thus, this chapter advocates that systematic attention be given to the people's own explanations of beliefs and practices invoked to promote health and prevent illness. Leininger suggests that knowledge of indigenous caring practices is the basis for health maintenance, recovery, and the prevention of illness, and is the foundation for providing nursing care that is congruent with local cultural traditions and lifestyles.[1]

Previous studies have focused on systems of folk illnesses and medical beliefs, and how these beliefs relate to the way people deal with illness.[2-7] This study examines those beliefs and practices deemed important to maintain health and prevent disease, with the assumption that such knowledge provides a holistic framework for planning and implementing primary health services, including nursing care.

THE SETTING

The setting for this investigation was a small *colonia* in a large highland city in Guatemala. The *colonia* contains 208 dwellings and is surrounded on three sides by a large ravine. A narrow bridge connects the *colonia* to the other portions of the city. A total of 1442 persons live in the small settlement. Residents are mostly Indian families, but there are some Ladinos.* There are no paved roads; most homes are made from adobe; many are without electricity and water. There is no sewage system: each home has an outside privy, while liquid garbage and waste materials drain onto the streets.

METHODS

A combination of approaches, including directed interviews, questionnaires, family health calendar recordings, and participant-observation, was used to collect the data for this study. Data were collected over a 13-month period, from November 1979 through December 1980. All interviewing was done in Spanish by the investigator, and the nature of the study was such that it provided an opportunity to study health and illness in families over a period of time within their natural environment.

The study population consisted of 22 households, or 134 individuals. A household is defined as a social unit containing either a single nuclear family (parents and children), or an extended family that is intergenerational and contains two or more mutually related nuclear families. The sample contained 11 single nuclear families and 11 extended families living as households of 2.4 nuclear families each on the average. Heads of sample households were identified as Indian (Cakchiquel), were born in the city where the study was conducted, and at the time of the investigation lived within the geographic boundaries of the *colonia*. All households in the sample were from the lower socioeconomic strata; average monthly income for heads of households was Q67.36 (US $67.36), a figure considerably below the minimum monthly wage of Q107.00 (US $107.00).

This chapter presents findings from the interviews designed to elicit data regarding beliefs and practices of self and family care. Members of the sample were asked to describe those practices that were believed helpful in taking care of themselves and that contributed to the good health of their family members. Analysis of the data revealed distinct categories which present a body of culturally relative knowledge that is the basis for health promotion and health maintenance in this cultural group. The practices that were described as important self- and family-care activities are shown in Table 10-1.

MAINTAINING AND PROMOTING HEALTH

Categories Relating to Hot-Cold

"Hot" and "cold" qualities, which have historically been attributed to Spanish classic medicine, are by far the most common conditions believed to influence health and illness in this population.[4] The qualities of hot and cold have no relationship to actual temperature but are ascribed states of various

---

*Ladinos are the Spanish-speaking majority in Guatemala. They are a racially and culturally varied group identified primarily by language and residence.

Table 10-1. A Guatemalan *Colonia* on Self and Family Care

Categories of Care-related Activities	Stated Goals
Avoidance of Environmental Threats and Personal Behaviors Related to Concepts of Hot-Cold	To Prevent Sickness To Have Good Health To Live Longer
Good Food and Regular Eating Patterns	To Provide Energy To Have Good Health To Prevent Weakness To Prevent Certain Diseases
Satisfactory Interpersonal Relationships	To Have Tranquility To Prevent Sickness To Enjoy Life
Sleep and Exercise	To Have Energy To Have Good Health
Good Work	To Provide for Family To Have Satisfaction For Socialization To Enjoy Life
Cleanliness and Personal Hygiene	To Prevent Disease To Have Good Health
Good Friends and Family Nearby	To Help When Needed To Enjoy Life

objects or persons. The notion of balance is intertwined with the concepts of hot and cold. Good health requires a balance or a maintenance of equilibrium between the two extremes. A person should not remain either "hot" or "cold" for too long. Statements of culturally important do's and don'ts were common in the data elicited. "Don't stay outside in the sun for a long time." "Don't go outside in the night air." "Don't get wet." "Wear warm clothing when it is cold outside." "Don't drink cold things." These were some of the most commonly expressed examples of self- or family-care activities the sample practiced to stay healthy.

Equally important, it is believed that a person should not change quickly from one temperature state to the other. For example, if a person has been walking outside and enters a house, he/she should not remove a coat or sweater right away. It is believed that the blood is "hot" and to "cool" it down quickly will result in susceptibility to illness. Tasks such as ironing or cooking cause the blood to heat; it should not be cooled down quickly by immediately going outside into the cold air. Mothers in the sample reported a reluctance to take ill children with fevers to doctors because the doctor would take off the "hot" infant's clothes and place a cold stethoscope against the child's chest.

Sample members see hot–cold aspects of the external environment as containing a variety of threats to their well-being; they must constantly recognize and deal with them. Rain, cold air, and the sun are the particularly prominent ones. Personal self-care practices can be utilized to minimize the harmful effects of external factors and, in turn, decrease individual susceptibility to illness. Therefore, a person may be admonished not to go outside in the cold (an external factor), but if necessary, coats, hats, or sweaters (self- or family-care activities) should be worn.

Good Foods and Regular Eating Patterns

The sample members believe that eating nutritious foods is an important way to maintain health and prevent illness. Foods viewed as nutritious are vegetables, meat, bread, eggs, and milk. Breakfast and lunch are viewed as the most indispensable meals. Dinner should be a simple meal, since one should not eat a great deal of food prior to going to bed. A typical breakfast consists of oatmeal with milk, bread, and bananas. Families with more economic resources have eggs two or three times per week. Lunch is usually soup with meat and vegetables or a meat dish served over rice. Dinner is sometimes only bread or tamales and coffee. Frequently, only coffee and tortillas are eaten for breakfast and dinner by very poor families. They are not viewed as particularly nutritious, only filling.

Along with eating nutritious foods, regular eating patterns are an important aspect of self- and family-care. Skipping meals is viewed as a bad habit that could lead to various kinds of illnesses. The sample members believe that food should be fresh, clean, and well-cooked. Food is usually consumed promptly after cooking; leftover food is seen as unsanitary and is thought to cause illness. Discussions of good eating habits were influenced by the notion of balance. Eating sufficient amounts of the right kinds of food is important; at the same time, one should not overeat.

Satisfactory Interpersonal Relationships

The individual's psychophysical state is believed to be extremely important in promoting health and preventing disease. Extreme anger, passion, grief, fright, anxiety, or sadness will render a person susceptible to illness. Beliefs regarding one's psychophysical state are related to the humoral classifications of strength and weakness. It is believed that emotions can cause physical symptoms of illness, and many explanations of self- and family-caring processes involve the strong-weak dichotomy from classic medicine.

The concept of strength is usually applied to people, but it can be applied to natural phenomena or inanimate objects such as food. A strong person is seen as an adult; men are considered stronger than women. Strong persons are able to work hard and do not suffer from illnesses; they are able by virtue of their strength to withstand heat, cold, exhaustion, and adversities. Children, because they are not fully developed, are viewed as weak; it is believed that they are more susceptible to illness and are unable to withstand severe threats to health.

Childbirth and menstruation render women weak, and they believe that special precautions should be taken during these periods for extra protection. "Strong" foods are avoided during menses, as are vigorous exercise, exhaustion, heavy work, and other factors that might further contribute to the weakened condition, such as getting too hot or too cold. Other conditions leading to weakness in both sexes are overexertion, sweating, hard physical labor, wounds, trauma, or any illness.

A person who is experiencing intense emotional states may become *muy fuerte* (very strong) and cause illness in others, or he may be weakened by his emotional state and become susceptible to certain illnesses. A "strong" person may inadvertently cause the symptoms of *mal ojo* (evil eye) in a child. Many of the traditional illnesses such as *bilis, susto,* and *colera* are associated with intense emotional states.

Bilis is probably one of the most frequently reported lay illnesses. It is caused by strong emotions of passion, anger, fright, or extreme sadness. *Colera*, which is caused by anger or other emotional upsets, is another term that is often used interchangeably with *bilis. Colera* is believed to be precipitated by quarreling, and in its extreme form may lead to a *desrame cerebral* (stroke) with resulting paralysis or death.

Doña Marta, a 72-year-old member of the sample, suffered from *bilis* caused by the worry of trying to keep up with her mischievous great-grandson, whom she tended while his mother worked. Doña Emelia reported that when her husband died, she experienced an attack of *bilis* so severe that she was unable to leave her house for more than six months. Doña Juanita complained of severe *colera* each time her eldest son stayed out late at night drinking. These illnesses were precipitated by emotional states but resulted in physical symptoms such as headaches, abdominal pain, nausea, and vomiting.

Strong emotions, especially anger, are seen as a kind of illness in some people and weaken them so that they are susceptible to other illnesses. Madsen suggests that such emotionally related illnesses occur more frequently in women in those societies that prescribe a limited role for women and in which strong expressions of emotion are not socially sanctioned.[8] During the time of this study, several women in the sample reported suffering from *colera* or *bilis*, whereas men did not. Informants generally agreed that men could become angry (*colera* or *enojado*), but that they usually did not become ill from the anger unless they were old and weak; then they might suffer a stroke. Madsen suggests that anger causes *bilis* in Tecospa Mexican women more often than it does in men because men can take out their frustrations by beating up a friend or a wife, or by getting drunk, which a woman may not do.[8] This appeared to be the case in the *colonia*, where alcohol indulgence and spouse abuse were common male behaviors, and *colera* and *bilis* occurred in the female population.

Sleep and Exercise

Getting the proper amount of rest and sleep is considered an important and necessary step toward good health. As a general rule, the sample members went to bed early, around 9:30 PM, and were up by 5:00 or 6:00 AM. Children need more sleep than do adults, and ill persons need extra hours of sleep and rest to recover from illnesses.

It is considered just as unhealthy to sleep too much as it is not to have sufficient amounts of rest. Sample members reported that the most healthful practice was to go to bed early, sleep well, and arise early in the morning.

Exercise is thought to be a self-care activity that is beneficial to health. Too much exercise or too little can be harmful. Working too hard can weaken the body and increase vulnerability to sickness. At the same time, prolonged inactivity can result in weakness and various debilitated states.

Good Work

The belief systems regarding work activities have several components. It is believed that work or, more specifically, having a good job is necessary for life satisfaction. Men reported that if they had a steady job which provided them with an adequate and regular salary, they experienced a sense of pride and satisfaction in knowing that they were able to provide well for their families. In this sense, they were able to fulfill the role expectations of father, husband, and provider. Men reported that lack of steady employment could result in anxiety, worry, tension, and concern, which could result in illness. Women reported that if unemployment was frequent or prolonged, the repercussions might lead to family dissension, alcohol abuse, or even to the break-up of the family.

The majority of women are employed in marginal economic activities such as domestic work or vending in the market. Although the amount of money they contribute to the family income is small, it is significant in the sense that often it is the woman's salary that is able to sustain the family during periods of financial crises. Thus, women too experience a sense of contribution to the support of the family. Women reported that they enjoy working outside the home. In a society that still restricts the role of women, a job provides a socially sanctioned means of meeting new people, making friends outside the family group, and socializing which is otherwise not available. These activities were viewed as being important components of a healthy life style.

In a more general sense, sample members reported that work is necessary for survival. Having regular work is the only way to ensure an income, which is used to obtain the basic necessities of housing, food, and clothing viewed as basic to good health.

Cleanliness and Good Personal Hygiene

For many mothers, close attention to cleanliness is the most important caring activity that they provide toward the good health of their families. These family care activities are viewed as a part of women's domestic roles and include keeping the house clean, preparing the meals, washing clothes, and seeing that children are bathed and washed regularly and that everyone in the family adheres to standards of personal cleanliness.

The material living conditions in the *colonia* present challenges to personal hygiene and sanitation. Women work long hours carrying water, washing clothes, and coping with an environment that is not conducive to cleanliness. Sample members believe that an unsanitary environment contributes to disease. The lack of a sewer system, unpaved roads, water shortages, contaminated foods, and the dust or mud (depending on the season) are viewed as contributory factors in the spread of disease. The general adherence to the scientific germ theory as an origin of disease is expressed by residents of the *colonia*. Life, to a great extent, is a constant battle against dirt, contamination, and disease inherent in the social and material conditions that exist in the environment.

Good Friends and Family

Members of the sample view the proximity in living quarters of other family members as an important contribution to the enjoyment of life. Family ties are close; the most common household composition is that of an extended family. The household compositions are structured in such a manner that the individual can draw upon the help and assistance of a broad spectrum of family members. The cooperation fostered by these residential patterns provides a basis for health promotion and maintenance activities as well as the care necessary in illness episodes.

Fifty percent of the sample families have close kin living in the *colonia* whom they see on a daily basis. All sample families have kin living in other parts of the city, and interactions with kin groups are frequent. Close friends are usually neighbors, schoolmates, or work or church associates. Data analysis of the social networks reveals that friendship ties are vital caring mechanisms in providing psychologic support when interpersonal crises occur.

In addition to the psychologic support and mutual enjoyment provided by the social networks of kin and friends, there is a practical advantage to having friends and family nearby. Families can be relied upon if one loses a job, becomes ill, or is a victim of other misfortunes. Families can provide food, shelter, and economic assistance. Friends can be a source of employment tips and small loans.

Extended social and kin relationships ensure social cohesion and contribute to the health and welfare of the group. The family perpetuates cultural traditions and helps to ensure continuance of familiar patterns of lifestyles.

Health behaviors are learned within the family constellation; the family system gives rise to learned behaviors and shared beliefs and values that promote health and prevent illness.

THE STRUCTURING OF INDIGENOUS CARING BELIEFS

Analysis of data related to self- and family-care activities which promote health and prevent illness has yielded sets of information that contrast significantly between categories. We can go beyond the specifics of the data in Table 10–1 and suggest the more general distinctions they represent. These distinctions are not derived in any strictly operational fashion from the data already presented, but represent a less formal, more abstract explanation of the findings. Table 10–2 shows the general distinctions in beliefs that are evoked to explain self- and family-care practices.

Table 10-2. Guatemalan *Colonia* on Health Beliefs to Explain Family Care Practices

External versus Internal Distinctions
Avoidance of Environmental Hazards
Balance
Interaction Between External Hazards and Internal Conditions
Strengths and Weakness in the Lifecycle
Age
Sex

There appears to be an overall external versus internal distinction, in which illness may result from contact with hazardous agents in the external environment, or from internally directed practices of an individual. This overall external versus internal explanation underlying health-illness beliefs has been described by Adams as an important feature of Mayan folk medical beliefs.[2] The actions that sample members take in attempting to avoid illness for the most part follow directly from their concepts of the causes of illness.

Self- and family-care practice relating to good health or the avoidance of disease is often guided by distinctions within the external-internal category. There is a generalized belief that contact with hazardous agents in the external environment should be avoided. These hazardous agents are usually defined on the basis of assigned hot-cold or strong-weak qualities.[4] In this regard, certain themes emerge which have been identified in diverse cultural groups. Snow has suggested that "the notion that the world is a hostile and dangerous place and that an individual is liable to attack from external sources is characteristic of the health belief systems of a great many people."[9]

Internally initiated changes in the body's state may also lead to illness. These changes are precipitated by the failure to maintain a healthful internal balance. There is good health in harmony, and danger in anything done in the extreme. Eating too much or not enough, staying out late at night, or getting too much sleep is bad for the body. Balance also exists in the concepts of hot-cold and strength-weakness, and again harmony and moderation are stressed.

Illnesses are also attributed to the interaction between the internal and external factors. An internal condition such as being too hot can predispose one to illness; the external hazard can be the cold air that actually precipitates the illness. Not wearing proper clothing in cold weather, or not refraining from sipping cold drinks or eating ice cream during hot weather, is an example of the interaction between internal and external factors. Those illnesses involving the action of an external agent upon the individual are often said to be a result of *descuido* (carelessness). These kinds of illnesses are thought to be preventable if the individual uses "good sense," exercises caution, or avoids the circumstances that lead to them.

Caring practices relating to health promotion are distinguished according to the life cycle of the individual. Particular illnesses are defined in terms of the nature of the sickness. This distinction is primarily a lay theory of illness causation. However, the sample members were also interested in the conditions and situations that led up to the illness so that they could avoid them or take precautions against the consequences. The age-sex differentials are associated with the concepts of strength and weakness, with strength related to the ability to withstand illness and weakness with increased vulnerability. Females are considered weaker than males, and this weakness is especially threatening during menses, pregnancy, or childbirth. Children are believed to be the weakest of all, a belief that is reinforced by the high infant mortality rates in Guatemala. Most folk diseases occur primarily in women and children. Cultural strategies for preventing folk maladies, such as the wearing of red ornaments by children, are common. Red is considered a "strong" color and is believed to offer children protection against *el ojo* (evil eye). The unborn child is influenced by his mother's prenatal behavior. Both men and women become weaker as they grow older and thus become more susceptible to illness. In these contexts, the life-stage of the individual is an important factor in self- and family-care activities. This distinction is one that has a general significance in health-promoting activities.

SUMMARY AND CONCLUSIONS

The self- and family-care activities and associated belief systems described in this chapter reflect a culturally based body of knowledge that contains the underlying rationales for actions taken to promote health and prevent illness.

Conceptions of health and illness are dominated by the "hot-cold" and "strength-weakness" theories, and behavior to promote health and prevent disease is in conformity with these beliefs. The belief that intense emotional states can produce illness was expressed by the sample; and precautions were taken to avoid or minimize illness due to such hazards.

On a more abstract level, several themes are evident in the data. First, the external versus internal distinction suggests that sample members see the external environment as containing a variety of threats to their health. The ability to identify sources of illness, however they are defined, is crucial, and failure to do so has potentially harmful results on one's health. The concept of moderation in everyday activities is interwoven throughout the expressed beliefs regarding healthful behavior and serves to guide daily life. Stages of the life cycle are believed to influence one's ability to withstand illness, and culturally sanctioned ways are defined to enhance, promote, and protect health during these crucial periods.

Beliefs and practices surrounding self- and family-care activities reveal a system of culturally defined knowledge that is aimed at promoting health and preventing illness. This shared knowledge is used in purposive action, since the behaviors instigated by sample members to avoid illness for the most part follow directly from these concepts.

REFERENCES

1. Leininger M: Transcultural Nursing: Concepts, Theories and Practices. New York, John Wiley and Sons, 1978.
2. Adams F: Un analisis de las creencias y practicas medicas en un pueblo indigena de guatemala. Instituto Indigenista Nacional, Publicaciones Especiales 17, 1952.
3. Foster GM: Relationships between Spanish and Spanish-American folk medicine. J Am Folklore 66:201–217, 1953.
4. Rubel AJ: Concepts of disease in Mexican-American culture. Anthropol 62(5), 1960.
5. Fabrega H: Towards a model of illness behavior. Medical care II(6), 1972.
6. Woods C, Graves TD: The Process of Medical Change in a Highland Guatemalan Town. Los Angeles, Latin American Center, 1973.
7. Young JC: Medical Choice in a Mexican Village. New Brunswick, NJ, Rutgers University Press, 1981.
8. Madsen W: Hot and cold in the universe of San Francisco Tecospa, valley of Mexico. J Am Folklore 68, 1955.
9. Snow LF: Folk medical beliefs and their implications for care of patients. Ann Intern Med 81:82–96, 1974.

11

Southern Rural Black and White American Lifeways With Focus on Care and Health Phenomena

"If the bottom of your foot itches, you will walk on strange land"; "Crowing hens will bring bad luck"; "You will have good luck if you throw a penny out the car window when passing a cemetery"; "Haste makes waste"; "Time and tide wait for no one"; "Beauty is only skin-deep—ugly goes to the bones"; "Aging can be beautiful and something to enjoy"; "If you care for people, you like this friendly place."

These folk statements provided the researcher with several clues about a different culture, namely, the southern rural Afro- and Anglo-American culture in the deep South. The author gradually discovered that if one cares for people, one will indeed like this friendly community in the South.

As a nurse-researcher interested in the systematic study and documentation of care and health values, beliefs, and attitudes of cultural groups, the author developed many new insights into the rural Afro-Americans (Blacks*) and Anglo-Americans (Whites) in south central Alabama. Their constructs of care, health, and ethnonursing practices were discovered.

The purpose of this chapter is to present some of the research findings from the investigator's study of southern rural Black and White cultures, with a focus on care and health values, beliefs, and practices, as well as on the general lifeways of the people. A full research report is being prepared on the cultures. Only major themes and findings are reported here.

---

*Throughout the chapter the term "Black" will be used as a shorthand expression for Afro-Americans and "White" for Anglo-Americans or Caucasians. These terms are used with the realization of their general limitations.

Besides studying the general lifeways of the people, the author investigated and analyzed several research questions in reference to her theory of the diversity and universality of transcultural care.[1,2] Some of the major research questions under investigation were:

1. What *ethnohealth (emic)* values, beliefs, and practices can be identified with the people?

2. What *ethnocare (emic)* values, beliefs, and practices can be identified with the people?

3. What are the perceived differences and similarities between the rural-folk and the urban-professional health care practices?

4. What is the general lifeway of the Black and White villagers, especially related to care and health cultural expressions?

5. What are the implications for therapeutic ethnocaring and ethnonursing care practices, based upon the research findings?

In this chapter, these questions are addressed in a general manner, with recognition that much more could be presented about the villagers.

DEFINITION OF TERMS

1. *Care:* refers to those assistive, facilitative, and/or enabling decisions or acts that aid another individual(s), group, or community in a beneficial way.[3]

2. *Health:* refers to beliefs, values, and action-patterns that are culturally known and are used to preserve and maintain personal or group well-being, and to perform daily role activities.

3. *Emic:* refers to the language expressions, perceptions, beliefs, and practices of individuals or groups of a particular culture in regard to certain phenomena.

4. *Etic:* refers to the *universal* language expressions, beliefs, and practices in regard to certain phenomena that pertain to several cultures or groups.

5. *Ethnocaring:* refers to the *emic* cognitive, assistive, facilitative, or enabling acts or decisions that are valued and practiced to help individuals, families, or groups.[2]

6. *Ethnohealth:* refers to those *emic* cognitive beliefs and actions preserve or maintain personal or group well-being, and to perfor role activities.

7. *Ethnonursing:* refers to *emic* learned knowledge, values, and practices of caretakers used to provide assistive, facilitative, and/or enabling actions or discussions beneficial to care recipients.

8. *Cultural care accommodations:* refers to cognitive-assistive actions and decisions or to plans to facilitate client-specific care that take into account the cultural beliefs, values, and practices of the client(s).

9. *Cultural care preservation or maintenance:* refers to those deliberative-assistive or facilitative actions or decisions that take into account ways to preserve or maintain cultural values and lifeways viewed as beneficial to care recipients.

10. *Cultural care repatterning:* refers to those deliberate actions that are assistive or facilitative to the client(s) and that combine several different aspects of a client's beliefs, values, or practices in a meaningful or beneficial manner.

11. *New cultural care practices:* refers to the cognitive action of incorporating different or new assistive or facilitative actions designed to be beneficial to the client.

THEORETIC AND CONCEPTUAL FRAMEWORK

The theory of transcultural diversity and universality of care and health was used for this study to describe, explain, and predict the lifeways of the southern villagers.[1] Essentially, the theorist holds that care and health differ with cultural cognitions, values, and practices among cultures, with some identifiable universal features. Social structure features (ie, religion, kinship, economic and cultural values) are closely related to health and care values and practices, and they influence or account for health care differences and similarities.

Culturally meaningful and efficacious nursing care is contingent upon the use of culturally derived ethnographic data on health and care. Ethnonursing is a culturally cognitive approach designed to be assistive and facilitative to individuals, families, and cultural groups in order to provide care that is congruent with clients' values, norms, and practices.[1] Ethnographic, ethno-logic, and ethnonursing data on cultures provide the bases for facts and principles of ethnonursing care practices. There are three major types of ethnonursing care and actions in therapeutic health practices: (1) care accommodations; (2) care preservation and/or maintenance; and (3) care repatterning. (See abovementioned definitions.) The theoretic and conceptual model that depicts these transcultural dimensions is found in Figure 11–1—the Leininger Sunrise Model—and has been discussed in other publications.[2,4] Other transcultural nursing care concepts, facts, and principles are available in other of the author's works.

Some major theoretic premises related to transcultural nursing theory are as follows:

1. Culturally based care values, beliefs, and practices are essential to human growth, living, and survival.

2. Care is the essence and the central, dominant, and unifying focus of nursing.

3. Health values, beliefs, and practices are derived from the culture, and vary between and within cultures.

4. Health and care concepts are identifiable by cultural groups and are linked together by cultural values and action patterns.

5. Features of social structure are powerful forces influencing health and care in any culture.

6. Folk *(emic)* and professional *(etic)* care and health values and action patterns are identifiable in a given culture.

7. Ethnocaring and ethnohealth concepts are essential for therapeutic ethnonursing care practices.

8. Care accommodations, preservation or maintenance of health, and repatterning are creative modes of providing ethnonursing care to achieve therapeutic outcomes, and are mainly based upon *emic* data of particular cultures.

9. Culture-specific and universal care practices can be identified and used as a sound basis for nursing care practices.[2,5]

The major hypotheses under consideration for this ethnonursing study are:

1. There is a close relationship between the social structure—including cultural values, practices, and beliefs—and ethnohealth and ethnocaring practices of cultural groups.

2. Rural folk and urban professional care practices reflect differences among people due to value differences regarding care and health.

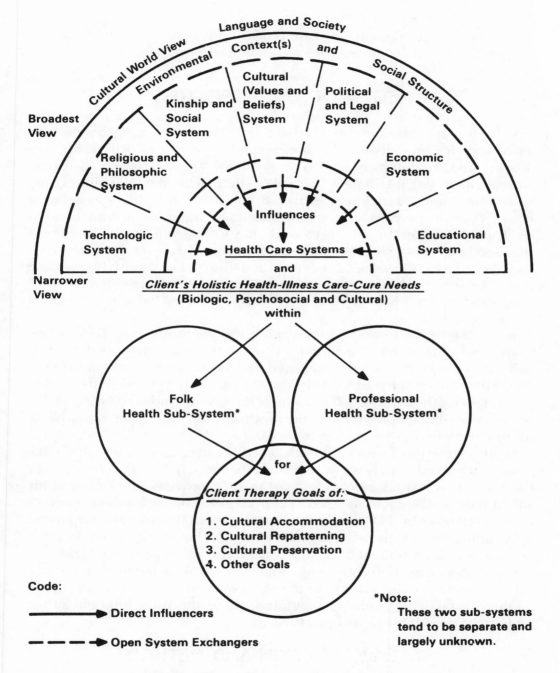

Focus: Individual, Family, Social and/or Cultural Group

Figure 11-1. Leininger's "Sunrise" Conceptual Model For Culturologic Interviews, Assessments, and Therapy Goals

3. The greater the differences between rural folk and urban professional care practices, the greater the need for nursing care accommodations and repatterning.

4. Therapeutic ethnonursing care is dependent upon the cognitive use of ethnocare and ethnohealth concepts, and ethnographic data.[5]

REVIEW OF THE LITERATURE

A review of the literature revealed that this was the first investigation focused on ethnocaring and ethnohealth lifeways of southern rural Afro-Americans (Blacks) and Anglo-Americans (Whites) in the United States. There are, however, many general reference books about the Black and White cultures from historic and contemporary perspectives. Billingsley's book, *Black Families in White America,* provides information about the interrelationships between Black and White families.[6] Lerner's work, *Black Women in White America: A Documentary History,* is another source of valuable data about Black women's lifeways and some of the social structures and historic factors influencing their lives.[7] Another publication that offers valuable cultural insights into Afro-American families is Stack's work, entitled *All Our Kin: Strategies and Survival in a Black Community.*[8]

Most recently, Kennedy's anthropologic research investigation, entitled *You Gotta Deal With It,* has provided a vivid description of many of the social, political, economic, and environmental factors influencing the health and illness status of southern Black Americans.[9] Kennedy cogently describes Black-White relationships influencing the general welfare and well-being of the people. The ethnographic findings are invaluable in grasping the Black-White cultural relationships in one area in the South.

Another study that focuses indirectly on ethnocaring and ethnohealth in the rural southern community is a work entitled *Becoming a Woman in Rural Black Culture.*[10] This investigation, completed in 1977, provides rich ethnographic and ethnologic data about adolescent maturation and the day-to-day lifeways of young Black women. The relationship between social structure and the process of becoming a woman is well presented. The study, however, does not focus on care and health, even though the author is a nurse and an anthropologist.

Although a number of other studies might be cited about the Black and White cultures, none pertains directly to the phenomena of care and health in the southern rural Black-White communities, or to the rural folk and urban professional health beliefs and practices.

RESEARCH DESIGN AND METHOD

The research was designed as an ethnographic, ethnologic, and ethnonursing study to describe and explain the health and care lifeways of a rural community in the southern United States. The design was for a 10-month field study of Afro-American (Black) and Anglo-American (White) villagers. In-depth interviews, participant-observations (with structured and unstructured interviews), life histories, daily living accounts, health care assessments, photographs, drawings, and other anthropologic and ethnonursing care methods and field techniques were used to study one community in an intensive manner. Qualitative and quantitative research methods were used as corroborative means to discover, describe, and validate the lifeways of the villagers. In the second village, a cursory study was done to obtain reflective comparative data to determine the "typical" aspects of the main community being studied. The ethnonursing and anthropologic research methods used in this study have been described in other literature sources and are not discussed here.[11-14]

VILLAGE DESCRIPTIONS AND SAMPLE

Two villages were chosen for the study. One village was chosen for an in-depth study and analysis, and is referred to by the fictive name of the Friendly Village. A second village was chosen to provide a *reflective comparison* with the Friendly Village to determine if the latter was highly unique. The second village was called Pecan Village. Friendly Village is the focus of this report, since it was the principal village studied intensively for approximately 10 months. Pecan Village is referred to occasionally for contrast. The researcher made regular visits to Pecan Village, but no in-depth ethnographic and ethnonursing study was done.

Both villages met the following criteria: (1) a southern village in a rural southwest central part of Alabama; (2) a small rural farm and town community linked to a moderately sized city (over 25,000 and under 50,000) within a 20- to 30-mile area; (3) a village with Afro-American (Black) and Anglo-American (White) people living together; and (4) a village perceived to be a typical rural southern village by indigenous people of the geographic area.

Friendly Village: The Major Research Focus

Friendly Village was a small town of approximately 2500 people located in south central Alabama. It was a town–farm community with about 300 people living in a 10-mile radius of the town. Most villagers saw the town and farms as contiguous. Approximately 60% of the villagers were Black (Afro-Americans) and 40% were White (Anglo-Americans)—approximately 1500 Blacks and 1000 Whites.

Historically, the town was established in the mid-nineteenth century by an interested White businessman. The town has always been dependent upon the rural crops, wood pulp, and small business enterprises. During the nineteenth century, cotton was the major crop until the boll weevil destroyed the plants. Today, peanut growing is the principal livelihood, along with the wood pulp industry and small businesses.

There are two schools: an elementary and a high school. There are two banks, 22 small stores, a police station, a small library, a fire and rescue station, approximately six gas stations, several auto repair shops, and about nine churches in the town and rural community. Unquestionably, the nine churches (two White-Baptist, two Presbyterian, and five Black-Baptist) were of central importance to the villagers. There is no hospital and only a small clinic, with one physician providing all professional health services. Three mortuaries (two used primarily for White people, and one for the Black villagers) and a home for the elderly are located in the village.

Black and White people tend to live in different geographic areas in the town, and they are interspersed in the rural community. Black and White villagers attend separate churches. The small businesses on the main street are mainly operated by White businessmen and women with assistance from Black villagers. The schools in the town are integrated; however, some White parents send their children to a nearby all-White urban School. Both Black and White people participate in business affairs and selected political, social, and religious activities.

In regard to economics, the yearly income for the average Black family (or household) was estimated by key informants (and from other data sources) to be approximately $5000-$7000 per year. There was great variability in Black and White incomes, in that 30% of the Black families and 5% of the White families had incomes of less than $5000 per year. There were no Black families known to have an income of more than $20,000 per year. Some White widows in the village were said to be both "wealthy and generous." The wide range of differences in family or household income made the lifeways of the people different, but cultural values seemed to play an even more significant role. Political, kinship, and religious aspects were major forces affecting the villagers' lives.

Sociocultural activities for White and Black villagers were largely influenced by religious beliefs and practices. Village activities that were initiated through the church seemed to be more acceptable and valued than nonchurch-based activities. Religious values were evident in business and social affairs. Many lifecycle ceremonial activities such as marriages, births, funerals, and teenage events reflected the sociocultural rhythm and daily patterning of the villagers' lives.

Pecan Village: A Reflective Contrast

Pecan Village, a reflective contrast, is a town–farm community with a population of 3000 people located in south central Alabama.

The Black to White population ratio in Pecan Village was similar to that of Friendly Village, ie, 60:40. Blacks and Whites lived in different geographic locations in the town and country, similar to Friendly Village.

Pecan Villagers mainly depend upon raising pecans, peanuts, and small grain crops. Wood pulp, general farm equipment, and several small-town commercial enterprises were other livelihoods. There were approximately 12 Baptist and

Presbyterian churches in the town and rural community—again similar to the Friendly Village in that they had nonintegrated church practices.

This village had a wide main street with several small clothing, grocery, drug, and appliance stores. The farm equipment and auto repair shops, along with the gas stations, were slightly greater in number than in the Friendly Village. Other businesses and community service shops found in Pecan Village were also found in the Friendly Village.

Religious activities were a dominant activity in Pecan Village, and were closely linked to social, economic, and political affairs—all features similar to the Friendly Village. The village's political council meetings with a mayor were held regularly. Church weddings were frequently held on weekends in the churches.

In general, the Pecan Villagers did not seem quite as friendly and ready to meet and accept strangers as the researcher found initially in the Friendly Village. Pecan and Friendly Villages had essentially the same social structure, and they knew the systems by which they functioned. Religious, kinship, and social aspects were slightly different in cultural expression and history, but the cultural values were similar.

Interestingly, both villages felt that they had a unique cultural history that made them different from other nearby rural and urban communities. However, the researcher found similar historic and migration patterns in the two villages. Slightly different lifestyles were identified, but common behavior patterns prevailed. When the researcher asked: "Do you have ways similar to or different from X village?" these statements were heard from the Friendly Villagers, who knew or had heard about Pecan Village: "They are not as friendly as our folks. We care for our people in lots more ways than they do. We raise more peanuts, fruits, and vegetables than they do and really care for each other around here." The Pecan Villagers said: "We have always been a friendly place. We raise more pecans, do more farming, and go to the 'big city' more than those folks."

Pecan Village was proud to have a 50-bed hospital serving the community, with approximately 22 nurses and 10 regular physicians. In addition, there was a 45-bed nursing home with adequate staffing.

As for location, Friendly Village was 10 miles from the nearby city with 30,000 people; Pecan Village was about 32 miles from this city. The villagers seldom interact with one another, and there is limited economic and social exchange. They know of each other only in name and in limited ways.

INFORMANT SELECTION

During the 10 months that the researcher interacted with many of the Friendly Villagers, she also met with a small number of the people in the Pecan Village. The researcher interviewed approximately 90 Friendly Villagers and selected 60 for in-depth study. The telephone directory was used to select every tenth villager for in-depth observations, interviews, and other research data. Two villagers informed the author whether the ones she had selected were Black or White so that she could get a 50% sample of the two cultural groups. The selection criteria for the Friendly Village were:

1. Adults and children who had lived in the village three years.

2. Southern Afro-Americans (Blacks) and Anglo-Americans (Whites).

3. Male or female villagers (approximately 50% of each).

4. Members of a family living in the community.

For the Pecan Village, the researcher did not use a random sample; instead, spontaneous "walk-up-to" or casual visits were made randomly. The researcher visited Pecan Village approximately three times each month for comparative reasons.

The researcher had no prior knowledge of either village, and there were no known formal anthropologic or ethnographic studies done in Friendly or Pecan Villages prior to this time.

ENTRY TO AND RESEARCH IN FRIENDLY VILLAGE

The researcher drove into Friendly Village and parked on a side street. Then she walked around to meet and visit with the people. As she drove into the village, she saw beautiful rolling hills, many forested areas, several small lakes, and plots of farmland. In one part of the village, there were painted and attractive large homes with well-kept yards. (She later found that these belong to Whites.) There were also unpainted, very small homes with fairly clean yards that belonged to the Blacks and poor Whites in the village. On one side of town, there were only a few White people seen working outside their homes, and very few children playing in the yards. In contrast, there were many children playing in the streets and yards where the Black people lived. During the day, about 10 to 20 people were usually found visiting or watching for someone, or both. Cars were driven down the highway or street in a slow and orderly way. Seldom were there teenage racers on the main or side streets.

A nursing student who attended the urban university about 10 miles away had recently moved into the Friendly Village with her husband and family. She suggested that the researcher might want to visit with a few persons who were leaders of the community. Among these persons was a man who was a leader of the Town Rescue Squad in Friendly Village. The researcher walked to his place of business and identified herself as a nurse and anthropologist who was interested in learning about the lifeways of this village, and especially how he thought the people kept well and prevented illnesses. She indicated to him (and others she met later) that she would like to visit and study the people during the next 10 months. He responded in a friendly way and said: "I think it would be good to study the villagers, since there has never been a study here." He then suggested other informants the researcher might visit to tell her about the people and their lifeways. He invited her back for a visit "any time."

From that initial visit and entry into the Friendly community, the author began to interact, observe, and participate in the community. Unfortunately, these rich experiences cannot be presented here, but will be reported later in another publication. In general, the ethnography and study of the people went well, with no major or serious problems. The author's previous studies of four other cultures enabled her to use her ethnographic and ethnonursing skills favorably, with considerable confidence and sensitivity to the people.

GENERAL REPORT OF FINDINGS

In this next section are reported some of the major findings and themes derived from study of the Friendly Village. The findings are of necessity briefly reported in relation to the research questions posed for this study.

Ethnohealth Findings

1. *What ethnohealth (emic) values, beliefs, and practices can be identified with the people?*

From the unstructured and structured ethnonursing interview guide, direct observations, and participatory experiences, several ethnohealth themes, values, beliefs, and practices were identified and discussed with the villagers.

1. Health had similar meanings for the Black and White villagers in that both viewed health as being "able to be up and around the place and able to do what is expected of you—that is, your business, garden, and house or job duties." This was manifested in their daily life practices by the "healthy man, woman, and child being able to work." The ability to be active in one's church activities was most important, and was most talked about in their daily work. The dominant theme abstracted from both Black and White villagers was the concept that *health means being able to do your work in the home, church, and community.* The villagers said that to be healthy, "one had to think about one's neighbors and friends and how one cared for or helped them." The criterion of being able to be *active* and to carry forth one's daily activities or role functions was stressed as being a desired value and norm of the villagers. For Blacks, the daily activities were mainly work in the garden and fields, and church activities. For Whites, being able to conduct one's daily business affairs at the store or on the farm was a determining factor of whether one was healthy. Hence, health was an objective reality, a practice, and of high value to the people, varying in degrees between Black and White villagers.

2. The *second* dominant meaning associated with health was *"to live by the Bible and do what Jesus (or God) teaches."* Ninety-two percent of the White and Black villagers would say: "If you follow what is in the Bible, you will be well and stay well." Practically all Black adults older than age 40 held firmly to the idea that religious beliefs and action patterns keep you well (98%). Many examples from the Bible were cited by Black villagers to substantiate that health and religion are tightly linked together, and that one cannot speak of health without considering the idea of spiritual health as a total way of living and acting. Black elderly people would say: "The Bible teaches you how to keep well and avoid evil thoughts and actions that could make you ill." One elderly man (age 93) said: "I don't think a lot of White (nonvillage) people understand health and the Bible. If they did, they wouldn't be running into that hospital (referring to the nearby city) for their children and themselves. One has to let Jesus be the healer. I have always let Jesus heal me when I get upset. I have never spent a day in the hospital, nor will I go there. Jesus can heal and keep you healthy. People who are not working with Jesus have to use other people to heal them." (This man was physically very healthy.)

The majority of the White villagers (85%) felt that religion was essential to remain well and "have presence." Many White Baptist and Presbyterian active church attendees frequently replied to the investigator's question "What makes you healthy?" with this reply: "I believe God keeps me well if I listen and pray to him. He knows how to get me well and keep us healthy in this community. I know this to be true." An older White woman (about age 91) said: "I rely on my friend or Jesus to keep me well. I have never been in the hospital. I read about those places." At church services, both Black and White villagers would often identify a list of 20 to 30 parishioners who needed Jesus (or God) to make them well. They would state each name and actively pray for keeping them well or for recovery from illness. White folks used the word "God" more frequently than "Jesus"; whereas the Blacks always used the word "Jesus" and the expression "Jesus heals and saves us—and always has."

Nearly 98% of all Black villagers belonged to the Southern Baptist fundamental religion. Adults and small children were regular church attendees; however, some of the young male teenagers (ages 14 to 30) did not always attend church on Sunday. Several told me that they "had work to do and Jesus did not do everything." Most White villagers (72%) attended the Southern Baptist churches, and the others attended the Baptist and Presbyterian churches. Salvation was with God or Jesus through *fellowship with others*, and by living together in the community in a concerned (caring) way. Doing what is right and avoiding evil can keep one healthy and well. These were themes from the White villagers.

The values of health, wellness, healing, and religion were inextricably linked together for both Black and White villagers. The concept of concern for others and self was often expressed as a healthy act, as well as visiting others when they were ill. While the villagers recognized sickness, it was more of a deviation from health (as described previously) and was not an isolated concept. *Sickness* meant the lack of a fully healthy person— a *wholeness* concept in fulfilling one's role and involvement expectations with others, ie, with families, individuals, community groups, and strangers.

3. The *third* idea associated with health was the means to *preserve* it: eating foods grown in one's own garden or raising foods that were viewed as good for them. They did not like to eat foods contaminated "by commercial solutions that the big city folks made, and put in tin cans." Many Black women and men proudly showed their canned (glass) food goods. Foods such as collards, peas (of 10 varieties), and turnips were particularly viewed as healthy for the Black villagers; whereas the White villagers saw lettuce, tomatoes, carrots, onions, sweet peas, and potatoes as *preserving* one's health. The concept of health preservation was linked with the caring value of concern. The villagers believed that if you are concerned about *others* (first) and then yourself (second), you will *preserve* good community health and your own health. The concept of focusing on others for self and community health was interesting.

Other concepts associated with health and the absence of health were expressed in response to this question: "What do you believe is unhealthy or not related to a good healthy lifeway?" The majority (94%) of responses were these: (1) "You are not being concerned about others" (Black or White villagers); (2) "You are not doing your work or job to keep healthy"; (3) "You are not understanding what Jesus tells us, and listening to and praying to Jesus, as he can make us well"; and (4) "You are unwilling to 'pitch in' and work or help others in this community."

ETHNOCARING FINDINGS

Turning to the villagers' responses to the question, "What ethnocare *(emic)* values, beliefs, and practices are identifiable with the people?", the following themes were revealed (Table 11-1). The villagers' responses were obtained by use of open-ended questions such as: (1) Tell me about your ideas of daily care; (2) Describe a caring person; (3) What does care mean to you and the people? and (4) What ideas seem most important about care?

The responses from 60 participants obtained through several in-depth interviews and recurrent sequenced daily observations by the investigator in the village are presented in Table 11-1. The comparative qualitative and quantitative data on the ethnocare values and meanings clearly show the domains of similarities and differences between the village cultural groups. Of interest is the

Table 11-1. Comparison of Care Meanings and Actions Among Black and White Friendly Villagers (60 Participants)

Black Villagers	Percentage	White Villagers	Percentage
1. *Concern for Others as Caring* (A) Providing for own "brothers'" and "sisters'" needs; (B) Being aware of others' needs; (C) Helping others to receive.	90	1. *Concern for Others as Caring* (Some self-care expressed) (A) Being aware of "friends'" needs; (B) Providing for "friends'" and self's needs; (C) Help/aiding others as a Christian.	93
2. *Presence as Caring* (A) "Being there" in need; (B) Being around the place or seen.	94	2. *Presence as Caring* (A) "Being seen around" here; (B) Being around village, church, job.	89
3. *Involvement as Caring* (A) Participate in family and neighborhood affairs; (B) Concern about one's "brother" or "sister."	76	3. *Involvement as Caring* (A) Participate in community affairs; (B) Talk and know happenings; (C) Participate in "fellowship" church activities.	92
4. *Touching One's Own "Brother"* (A) In time of sorrow and losses; (B) To know reality as it is; (C) To elicit true family feelings.	97	4. *Selective Touching as Caring* (A) On special occasions; (B) As act of affection or to help others.	18
5. *Sharing as Caring* (A) Sharing food among family; (B) Sharing through religious experiences; (C) Sharing to survive; (D) Sharing as a family responsibility.	89	5. *Sharing as Caring* (A) Sharing food, goods, information, and money with others; (B) Sharing through religious fellowship activities; (C) Sharing social and religious experiences.	92

Table 11-1. *(Continued)*

Black Villagers	Percentage	White Villagers	Percentage
6. *Caring with Sex Role Differences* (A) Mother as main caregiver and provider in home; (B) Father as providing care through external resources; (C) Religion ascribes sex roles and care practices.	76	6. *Caring with Sex Role Differences* (A) Mother as child caregiver; (B) Father as "material goods" provider; (C) Religion ascribes sex role differences.	84

fact that the *emic* care values could be identified and described by the villagers once this area of inquiry was made known to them. Hence, *cognitions of care were identifiable and could be explained by the people.* Some of the domains of similarities and differences in care are discussed next with their meanings and beliefs.

First, care meant *concern for others* for the Black (90%) and for the White villagers (93%). Both saw concern for others as most important, but some White villagers would also include concern for self. Repeatedly the Black and White villagers said: "We have always been concerned for one another since we first came here over one hundred years ago." "Concern" translated to the villagers as being interested in others and being helpful to people in the community. One woman villager (age 32) had gone to live in California and returned to visit her family. When I asked her about similarities and differences in living and health maintaining, she quickly replied: "Oh, it is so good to be back home in this community. These folks really care for you and are concerned about you. In California, they don't care one bit for you and everyone is for themselves. I also miss these Friendly Villagers. Here, everyone is concerned about each other and helps one another." A Black woman in the group said, "I have always lived here and I'm fixin' not to leave. We folks know how to care for one another. I depend on the White folks and they depend on me. If I needed help, I would go to my close Black and White friends, and they would help me." Many Black women and men made similar statements. Concern was also expressed by 90% of Black villagers in these ideas: Concern means (1) being aware of friend or community needs; (2) providing for one's own "brothers" and "sisters" in a religious and cultural way in order to help them survive; and (3) helping others who need care to accept and receive it. With respect to the latter, several Black villagers told the investigator that it is difficult for some Whites to receive care (or help) because of their pride. The Blacks said that they teach their families how to receive care in order to survive.

The White villagers spoke about concern for others in a way similar to the Black villagers; however, subtle differences from the Blacks existed. For Whites, care means concern for others, especially as Christian friends and friends in need. They explained that care is a human need, for often there are limited human and material resources, and one must care for friends. Other ideas associated with care and validated by practice were: (1) Providing *direct* help to "friends" in need under stressful conditions when they are helpless or feel helpless (note that White villagers use the term "friend," which is different from the more common Black term of "brother" or "sister"); (2) being helpful toward others as an expectation of Christian fellowship; and (3) showing concern by getting actively *involved* in assistance for others in need.

Interestingly, both Blacks and Whites view care as an *activity* and a *necessity* for health. Care as healthy concern is closely linked with being active and helping others. The idea of "watching out for" or "pitching in" to help someone in need was frequently stated by the Black and White villagers. Historically, the villagers gave many examples of the Blacks helping the Whites with their work for many decades on the farms and in town. Reciprocally, the Whites said that they often helped the Blacks with money, food, equipment, and so forth. Both types of villagers are afraid, with forced integration and outside influences, that this reciprocal helping process, value, and lifeway between Blacks and Whites will be lost. They firmly stated that "we knew how to care for each other as a decent White family and Black individual or family" through the years.

Through ethnoscientific analysis, other differences regarding care were identified. Care for the Black villagers was unequivocally related to survival, whereas the Whites saw care as preservation and as always being attentive to friends' or others' needs or losses. Furthermore, for the White Baptists, care was a "Christian act" (ethical) that should be valued and continued.

Two White bank managers (who have been in the villages many years) spoke about care as concern for others. They said that they always cared for Blacks by lending them money or credit in times of need. They knew Black families, and trusted and worked with them. For nonvillagers, it was much more difficult to get quick bank credit or money unless they were linked to the Church through family or friends. Anticipating needs of Black or White villagers was important and a desired cultural value to be preserved. Exploitation between Blacks and Whites was denied when this topic was pursued.

The *second* major ethnocare concept identified through ethnographic study was *presence* as *caring*. Both the Black (94%) and White (89%) villagers in the Friendly town and farms identified presence as caring. The people defined *presence* as *making a direct personal appearance or remaining with another villager as a sign of care*. Several villagers said: "If you care for others you will be with them. You will come and see others in person. You will show your concern by your presence. This means a lot to us." One Black man said: "If you are concerned and care for people, you come around here. We see them. They know they can get help from us—and we help them. If they don't come, then we aren't caring—we can't do too well without their being here."

Presence was more important for the Black than the White villagers. Presence is validated by "seeing you at church, seeing you at business, seeing you at the home place." said Black women. Many Black teenagers and grown adults held that being present at the annual church homecoming is extremely important to being a caring family and church. Hence, presence at the Annual Baptist Homecoming was imperative and a test of *presence as caring*. Black villagers save money and make great sacrifices to come home each year for this church and family homecoming. The Blacks repeatedly said that when there's sickness or death, it is important that a family member *be present*. Then one is a caring and concerned person.

For the White Friendly Villagers, *presence as caring means "being seen around" the home and community or at one's place of work*. It also means "being around" so villagers can see that one is all right or needs help. One cares for and prevents illness problems. Presence at church social gatherings or fellowship nights is an important means of validating presence as caring. As several villagers said: "If you are not present at these church meetings, or not seen around, we are concerned." Presence for Black and White villagers was an extremely important component of care, with ethical implications for Black families, and socioreligious expectations for White villagers.

The *third* dominant ethnocaring component of the Friendly Village was *involvement as caring*. Seventy-six percent of the Black villagers and 92% of the White villagers held that involvement was important to caring. For the Black villagers, involvement meant *participating directly in activities to assist others*. The major indicators that validated involvement as caring were: (1) participating in Black extended-family affairs for a variety of reasons, ie, getting food, clothing, or information, or doing general work activities for survival; (2) actively discussing affairs affecting one's Black "brother" or "sister"; and (3) using one's religious beliefs and kinship values to help Black and White people. Several detailed ideas about involvement were abstracted from the raw ethnographic and ethnologic data. This reflects the emphasis and the variety of ways that one can, and should, be involved as a Black villager.

Ninety-two percent of the White villagers identified involvement as caring and defined it fairly similarly to the Black villagers. There were, however, differences in the ways one becomes involved in the various kinds of activities. For example, ethnoscientific analysis of data revealed that these forms of involvement were important: (1) participating in community affairs; (2) being involved in different church and work activities; (3) participating as a caring person by talking about village happenings with others; and (4) being a Christian in its sense of involvement with others.

The *fourth* concept of caring was physical and psychosocial *touching*. Touch was culturally perceived and experienced as part of caring, but showed cultural variations among the villagers. Ninety-five percent of the Black villagers held that "touch" means placing one's hands on another person with different degrees of firmness or lightness depending on the occasion or need of the person. The form and variation of touch as body-to-body contact varied. Several Black villagers said: "We have always used touch to care for our 'brothers' and 'sisters,' in times of sadness and happiness." Touching to them was an important cultural expectation from birth through death. It was viewed as "a way of feeling and knowing how things really are. It is to let our family know that we are fully there in a real way." The researcher observed Black mothers stroking the newly born infant by rubbing the soles of the infant and touching every part of the body. The touching was done gently and with a smile on the mother's face. Black women and girls say they do much more touching of one another in crisis and noncrisis situations than do men and Whites. The researcher observed women and girls putting their arms around each other, rubbing arms, or engaging in spontaneous body (torso) embraces. Black people touch on joyous and sad occasions. They give upper-body hugs and firmly clasp hands on the death of a loved one or on a happy occasion. With the loss of homes, cars, or money, touching by a shoulder embrace was often seen in the Village. At funerals, the investigator witnessed much body touching, hand clutching, and mouth and cheek kissing. The dead person was touched at the mortuary and at the church services by Black family members and friends.

In marked contrast, White villagers did not touch one another as often as Blacks (only 18%). There were more cultural taboos about the unspoken "proper" time, place, and occasion to touch. Their touches were much less spontaneous, more formal, and more reserved. Occasionally, the researcher observed some handshakes between White adults, but only on special occasions or when they had not seen each other for a period of time. Strangers (nonvillager) usually offered their hand before the White villagers offered it. Handshakes as ritual greetings were acceptable on the streets, at the farm home, and at ceremonial events. Occasionally, kisses on the mouth and body embraces were observed among Whites, but they were much more reserved than among Blacks.

The amount of touching between Whites and Blacks was interesting in both the Friendly and the Pecan Villages. In the past, there was an unspoken cultural *taboo* for Blacks and Whites *not to kiss*, hug, or intimately touch one another except on very rare occasions, and then it was not in public. Today, this cultural norm generally prevails, but not entirely, since some Black and White adults were observed to give hugs on a few occasions. Black informants said: "We just don't touch or give a handshake unless the White person offers his (her) hand first. While we feel close to some, we would like to touch them, but don't." One middle-aged Black said, "It will take time, but I hope it happens some day, as true brothers and sisters." Several villagers were pleased and surprised that the researcher "offered your hand so quickly and were not afraid to sit on our porches and in our houses." They continued, "Most Whites seem afraid to touch us and visit with us in our homes. They are good to talk with us in the banks, business, and their homes. We get along fine and respect each other, but don't touch much." White villagers did not seem aware of the value of touching Black villagers, but they were aware of the cultural norms.

Several older Black women who raised and cared for children expressed concern that "young girls do not spend as much time touching the infants as they did in the past." The Black women believe that "touching (stroking) the infant a lot, from birth until they can run about, is an important part of caring for the child. It helps them grow healthy." They added, "We want this good child care practice to continue into the future and are trying to teach them how to touch infants when they have children."

White nurses working in Pecan Village were aware that Blacks, while in the hospital, touch their infants and clients more often. The nurses said, "This was hard for us to do, as we White nurses have not seen that need in the past." Several said it was easier to touch the Black children than teenagers and adults. As the researcher explored the idea, the White nurses became more cognizant of touching Blacks and of their feelings about psychocultural and physical touching.

These ethnocaring components of concern, presence, involvement, and touch were discovered from direct observations and interviews. Differential features were noted in the ethnonursing and domain analysis. Several additional features were noted which appeared important between Whites and Blacks, and which were areas generally not heretofore documented and talked about by the villagers. Each care construct was extremely relevant to care and cure processes.

RURAL AND URBAN FOLK PROFESSIONAL HEALTH CARE

With respect to the question, "What are the perceived differences and similarities between the rural folk and urban professional health care practices?" several findings became evident. They are briefly highlighted here. Rural folk and urban professional lifeways could be markedly contrasted by direct observation and through the viewpoints of the Black and White Friendly Villagers. Table 11-2 shows some of the major areas of comparative differences among the Friendly Villagers as well as their first-hand experience with the nearby urban community. Oral legends and folk tales also were heard concerning these differences.

1. The rural folk lifeway was viewed by 96% of the Black and White villagers as "the best and most secure lifeway." They saw the urban lifeway with health professionals as less desirable, and they feared going to the urban hospital because there were "potential dangers and evils." The rural villagers on the farm and in the town could quickly identify why they preferred staying in their own location. Several villagers had gone to moderate (over 25,000) and large cities (over 100,000), but they soon returned. More than 72% said they were very frightened while in these cities and got confused and disoriented. It was clear that the larger the city and the further away from home they went, the greater the tendency to become confused and disoriented. Several teenagers and adults (20 to 30 years of age) had "tried" going to large cities to visit relatives or friends, and told the researcher, "I am glad to be back home where it is safe and secure. Those people are not friendly like we are here. They don't trust anyone; they stare at you, take your money, and never say 'thank you.'"

Several Black and White adult men and women of the village frequently mentioned many accounts and legends about going to a nearby urban hospital to get professional help. They said, "The further I got away from here, the more frightened I became. While the hospital staff is nice, you still are in a strange and frightening place. You are a number. They quickly get information and your money from you, but we don't know them." Another man said, "I signed more papers than I ever did my whole life—and I was confused the whole time I was there. Do tests show confusion as expected behavior?" Several were frightened as they were told

Table 11-2. Cognitive Differences Between Rural Folk and Urban Professional Health Care of the Friendly Villagers (60 Participants)

Rural Folk Health Care Lifeways	Urban Professional Health Care Lifeways
1. The best and most secure lifeway (96% of both Black and White villagers).	1. A frightening experience with potential dangers and "evils" for rural folks.
2. A friendly and healthy way of living: (A) Friends and families care for each other; (B) Friends care for and heal each other.	2. Friendly in hospitals with: (A) A few family and friends; (B) No support and alone; (C) Confusing the further away from home.
3. Rural home remedies are helpful (Blacks 95%; Whites 56%).	3. White doctors spend all their time diagnosing and doing treatments of bones and body. Personnel do not see villagers as "whole persons" (Blacks 90%; Whites 62%).
4. Religion helps heal and is used in rural lifeway (95% of both Black and White Villagers).	4. Religion is limitedly practiced in the city.
5. Local caretakers and healers.	5. Strangers attempt to give care in ways strange to rural folks.
6. Know foods and activities that keep rural people well and healthy.	6. Urban people eat canned foods in tins, which are artificially preserved and not good for them.
7. Can get immediate care and help, if needed.	7. Have to sit for hours in hospital waiting room for help when really ill.
8. Cost is known, modest, and reasonable.	8. Cost of hospital services is very high.
9. Like to stay at home, and be with folks rather than with strangers in unknown and strange place.	9. Tend to get frightened when leaving the rural area. ("People unknown are impersonal and cold.")
10. Talk the same way and understand each other.	10. Talk different with lots of strange words and strange actions.

Table 11-2. *(Continued)*

Rural Folk Health Care Lifeways	Urban Professional Health Care Lifeways
11. More signs of being well if live at home (rural) environment.	11. More signs of illness, crime, and social problems in the city.
12. Quiet and peaceful in rural area.	12. Noisy and dirty in the city.

to go from one place to another and to follow lines on the floor and signs. Several disliked waiting in the hallway for hours.

Several Black villagers (of all ages and both sexes) were frightened by the urban experience, and said they hoped they would not become ill. It was too frightening to them because "those folks (urban doctors and nurses) don't know our talk and ways." They concluded, "It's best to stay at home and live with your aches, broken bones, or internals that don't work, rather than go to that strange place (hospital)." Most of the Black villagers older than 50 years said they preferred to have local women care for them, or to have care "from our own known physician in this town." The Black villagers use a number of local folk medications and healing practices that have long been used by the Black southern folk healers and carers—most of the care administered by mothers and grandmothers. Their practices are passed on through oral traditions and demonstrations to younger female adults. The use of kerosene for injuries and dermatitis and the use of a variety of local salves and massage treatments are common for Black folk carers and curers.

Both the Black and White villagers are pleased with the local male physician. He is a native to the community and listens to the people, and he does not demean their local treatments. The researcher found the villagers (over 90%) thought of the White physician as helpful and one who could be trusted. The physician told the researcher, "They know what helps them, and some things tend to work, so I let them go ahead and use them." Because of his good rapport with and trust of the Friendly Villagers, this physician has been giving medical services to the people nearly 50 years. In general, the villagers trust and value the physician and how he helps them. The author found that none of the villagers disliked this physician's services, and that he has integrated folk and professional services in an effective and sensitive way.

2. Several villagers said they disliked most professional ways in the urban hospitals and clinics because they are not treated as "whole people" and because of the "unfriendly folks." The emphasis on physical problems is different in that their view of being a whole person involves their religious, family, and other beliefs and values. When they are in the urban area, they often have no one near to support them because their family and friends cannot remain with or near them while in the hospital. This leaves them insecure and at risk with the urban professional staff. They also said that when they had to go to the "big hospital" and the "big city," they had to leave their family and friends behind—people that knew them and how to care for them. The Blacks disliked waiting around for hours because they had to leave their children and elderly family members at home alone. One Black man summarized the hospital experience as, "You are without your family and friends. There is no one to care for you like we do

in this community. We like our small doctor's office here in this community. He's safe and he knows us."

3. The majority of the Black (95%) and of the White villagers (56%) perceived that the rural life was best because they knew that home remedies were effective and because they had direct control over the use of these home remedies. In the urban hospital and community, these home remedies seemed to be unknown, and cure was totally controlled by the health personnel. Several feared the power of professional medicines compared with their home remedies. Ninety percent of the Black villagers and 62% of the White villagers found that the professional physician seemed mainly interested in diagnosing an illness, but did not help one keep well. Nurses did more in this area.

White villagers were much more tolerant of medical diagnostic and treatment regimens than the Black villagers. Some White villagers wanted to try new medicines and treatments, but would trust only a few. The Whites and middle- and upper-class villagers viewed going to the "big city" and to specialists as prestigious, and they were willing to pay for such services. They did, however, note the absence of a warm and friendly attitude on the part of the health professional toward them. Dependency on and control by the "big city" physician was evident. At the same time, many White villagers valued the use of modern technology such as cardiac resuscitation and the latest heart revival equipment. The Village Rescue Squad was mainly a team of White villagers who valued modern equipment and perfecting their skills.

4. Rural lifeways incorporate and allow for their religious and kinship beliefs and practices, whereas in the big city, these are absent. They perceive this as a major lack in urban professional services that needs to become part of healing, diagnoses, treatment, and care practices. Practically all villagers (more than 95%) wanted religion to be used in healing, curing, and caring for the people, and the Blacks wanted the extended family to be active participants in health care.

5. The Friendly Villagers said, "I know who can help me get well at home, but I am not sure who can help me when I go to that big (more than 60 beds) urban hospital." They acknowledged that lots of special equipment and experts are used, but they still do not know what works and why. The "magic" or urban practices were part of the perception of health care— and a disturbing factor. The adolescents were, however, curious about the "city hospital things and ways." The Black villagers didn't know if they could trust White strangers that they don't know. Adolescent boys had several "weird stories" about what folks do in the big city. In general, the urban professionals are strangers, as is the environment in which they

work. It is a risk of great concern to the Black villagers, but of considerably less concern to the White villagers.

6. The Black villagers were concerned that the nearby hospital did not provide the foods that they believed were healthy for them. While hospitalized, they may or may not receive foods such as chicken and bean soups, collards, and other southern foods. The older Black villagers would request their families to bring these foods to them (if they could sneak them in). The White villagers were not as concerned, but did value their beans to help them get well. Naturally raised garden foods were much preferred to the canned foods, as the latter are often perceived as "poisonous" by the Black villagers.

Other points of contrast can be noted in Table 11-2; several of these contrasts between rural and urban perceptions are comparable to other cultures studied.[15] Blacks communicating with Whites was of major importance, as was assessing attitudes of Whites in urban environments regarding their friendliness or hostility. Rural Blacks find that White people talk "strange," and Whites may find it difficult to understand them, since southern Black language is different from Anglo-American. A major finding was that the greater the distance away from the village, the greater the signs of fear, anxiety, and confusion in rural adult Blacks, especially in regard to what might happen to them in an urban hospital. For them, an urban hospital poses greater risks. The implications of this predominant finding must be given consideration by nurses, physicians, and other health care providers.

IMPLICATIONS FOR ETHNONURSING CARE

To address the question, "What are the implications for ethnocaring and ethnonursing care practices?", several points can be made in this last section. One of the most important implications is the realization that meaningful and therapeutic nursing care judgments, decisions, and actions should be based upon cultural data derived from cultural values and social structural knowledge. The social structural framework provides the most comprehensive and holistic perspective for knowing and understanding human health and caring behavior.[4] A second important principle derived from this research is the realization that care and health can be cognitively identified and documented by ethnonursing research methods and techniques. Ethnocaring and ethnohealth data derived from the client, family, or cultural group provide essentially new data (*emic*) for understanding and helping clients *from their viewpoint* and from the world view rather than relying so heavily upon professional (*etic*) assessments, judgments, and knowledge.

From the research findings of this study, the following implications for therapeutic ethnonursing can be offered:

1. Ethnocare and ethnohealth constructs of *concern*, *presence*, *involvement*, and *touch* were dominant values and practices of the southern rural Black and White villagers in the United States. These values are facts to guide therapeutic care.

2. Health and care for the Black and White rural villagers had similar meanings and values, but there were also differences in the cultural and psychosocial forms of expression. Hence, cultural similarities and variabilities were identified.

3. Cognitions, perceptions, and experiences related to rural folk and urban health professional views about health care services and experiences reflected marked differences from rural-folk Blacks' concerns, fears, and confusions about urban health professional attitudes and practices in a city hospital. White rural villagers had more favorable perceptions and experiences. Black and White male teenagers revealed mixed acculturation, with an attitude of curiosity toward the city hospital.

4. Several areas of cultural conflict and stress exist between Black rural folk and the predominantly Anglo-White urban professional health system, which necessitated cultural care accommodations or repatterning of urban health services, or both, to fit the cultural needs, values, and concerns of the people.

5. The concept of touch as a caring value, belief, and practice reflected differences between the Black and White rural villagers. It requires specific nursing care accommodations.

6. Specific care practices need to be developed to provide *culture-specific* care for the Friendly Villagers, with slight variations in the nursing interventions related to *presence*, *involvement*, and *concern*.

7. Use of other specific care and health findings from this study need to be explicated for greater precision and for provision of meaningful care to the villagers.

The interrelationships between care and health in the Friendly Village social structure and values are under full analysis, but are not reported here.

In summary, this was an ethnographic, ethnologic, and ethnonursing investigation of southern rural Afro-American (Black) and Anglo-American (White) villagers over a 10-month period. It focused on ethnocare, ethnohealth, and general lifeways of the people. The partial findings reported in this chapter indicate the importance of identifying care and health values of cultures from an *emic* perspective. This research study is part of a larger transcultural care study of a number of Western and non-Western cultures. Cultural differences prevail among most of the 30 cultures studied, and only a few common care constructs were universal (*etic*) among the cultures studied.[3] More systematic and in-depth investigations of specific cultures are needed to verify and validate caring and health cross-culturally. Moreover, similar ethno-methodologies need to be considered for their reliability and validity factors.

From this study, however, health personnel could initiate specific nursing care interventions to help the community maintain favorable health care practices. Most important, the study points to the need to base health and care practices upon the clients' perceptions, cognitions, and experiences, rather than impose health professional practices and ideologies on representatives of different cultures, so that meaningful and satisfying health services can be realized.

REFERENCES

1. Leininger M: Transcultural Care Diversity and Universality: Theory of Nursing. (*in press*.)
2. Leininger M: Transcultural Nursing: Concepts, Theories and Practices. New York, John Wiley & Sons, 1978.
3. Leininger M: Caring: An Essential Human Need. Proceedings of the Three National Caring Conferences. Thorofare, NJ, Charles B. Slack, Inc., 1981, p 9.
4. Leininger M: Intercultural interviews, assessment and therapy implications. *In* Pederson, P (ed): Interviews and Assessments. Beverly Hills, CA, Sage Publishers, 1981.
5. Leininger M: Caring: a central focus for nursing and health care services. Nursing and Health Care 1(3):135–143,176, 1980.
6. Billingsley A: Black Families in White America. Englewood Cliffs, NJ, Prentice-Hall, 1968.
7. Lerner G (ed): Black Women in White America: A Documentary History. New York, Random House, 1970.
8. Stack C: All Our Kin: Strategies for Survival in a Black Community. New York, Harper and Row, 1970.
9. Kennedy TR: You Gotta Deal with It: Black Family Relations in a Southern Community. New York, Oxford Press, 1980.
10. Dougherty MC: Becoming a Woman in Rural Black Culture. New York, Holt, Rinehart, and Winston, 1978.
11. Spradley J: The Ethnographic Interview. New York, Holt, Rinehart, and Winston, 1979.
12. Pelto RJ: Anthropological Research: The Structure of Inquiry. Intentions and Theory of Anthropology. New York, Harper and Row, 1970.
13. Spradley J: Participant-Observation. New York, Holt, Rinehart, and Winston, 1980.
14. Leininger M: Ethnonursing research field methods: a different approach to traditional research in nursing. (Unpublished paper, 1981.)
15. Leininger M: Transcultural nursing: its progress and its future. Nursing and Health Care. New York, National League for Nursing, September, 1981.

12

Gender-Related Perceptions of Caring in the Nurse-Patient Relationship*

Nurses generally agree that care is an important aspect of the nurse-patient relationship; however, disagreement exists among nurses regarding the importance of care behaviors in the relationship. Furthermore, nurses have been unable to agree upon a definition of caring and the unique features of care that are the historic basis for nursing practice.

The goal of establishing nursing as a profession within the health care delivery system has not been achieved, but the solution to this major problem may be found in the explication of care as the major focus of nursing. Moreover, the identification of caring behaviors in the nurse-patient relationship may well be the quality that defines nursing's unique contribution to health care systems.

CARE: IMPORTANT TO NURSES AND NURSING

The terms "care" and "caring" are often associated with child-rearing, interpersonal closeness, and personal relevance, and very frequently are used in references to nursing education and practice. The terms lack specific meaning, but they are relevant to health practices. Still, today care is viewed by many as less important than curing.[1-3] Leininger holds that the concept of caring is central and unique to nursing practice and education, and her research, teaching and leadership efforts reflect her commitment to care.[4] The past five National Research Caring Conferences for nurses and others interested in caring have opened the door to explore in depth the concept and meaning of care. In fact, the Conferences have been directed at the following: advancement of the body of

---

*Edward Murray, MA, PhB, was consultant for the research design, questionnaire, and data statistical manipulation.

knowledge upon which care is based, explanation of caring in relation to nursing, investigation of care behaviors from a transcultural perspective, and stimulation of persons to investigate care phenomena systematically.[5]

Investigation of care and caring behaviors relative to nursing is imperative for nurses as well as for nursing. Because the concept is widely used yet lacks specific definition of behaviors, one must ask if nurses can remain loyal to this illusive concept. Can nurses who make claims to care as part of nursing be accepted in health services without more knowledge about care? What do nurses know about client perceptions in nurse-patient relationships?

The study of interpersonal nurse-client care presents difficulties not encountered in the technologic cure-oriented arena. Ray points out, in an essay presented at the First National Research Caring Conference, that the emphasis that has been placed upon quantification methods to test hypotheses has not resulted in an identified underlying general thesis for nursing. Based on this lack of an underlying foundation for nursing knowledge, Ray developed and presented a philosophic analysis of caring in nursing.[2]

Because the term "care" is used so widely by individuals and groups of nurses in practice and education settings, it is imperative that nurse-researchers scientifically quantify the largely philosophically analyzed and accepted, illusive qualities known as care and caring phenomena.

REVIEW OF THE LITERATURE

There is an abundance of articles in the literature addressing the importance of and the need for caring in the nurse-patient relationship, but few are research studies. Furthermore, the articles and studies that focus on caring vary in purpose and direction. A number of articles talk about attributes of nurses and their general behavior without systematically investigating care. A few of these articles are cited here.

Goldsborough spoke of nursing in terms of involvement that is sharing feelings, ideas, beliefs, and values with the patient. She identified three ways that the nurse shares feelings with the patient, namely: (1) creating an atmosphere in which the patient feels free to express his feelings, (2) accepting the patient as a person who has the right to free expression, and (3) actively seeking to understand why the patient feels the way he does and helping him become aware of and understand his feelings.[5]

Velazquez found that nurses do not listen with all their senses to what patients tell them. She proposed that nurses who listen become involved in caring and committed to providing quality nursing service. Velazquez extended the notion that because they care, these nurses enlarge their participation in cure.[6]

In an interview by Harlem, Hall stated that since "cure" is considered much more progressive than "care," particularly in the developed countries where advances in medical technology have been tremendous, nursing and nurses have a primary responsibility for the much-needed development of care.[1]

Mayeroff identified and described eight major ingredients of caring: (1) knowing and understanding the other's needs both generally and specifically, (2) alternating the rhythm of help based on maintaining or modifying behavior, determined by judgment, (3) patience in giving an opportunity to the other to find himself, (4) honesty regarding a genuine openness with oneself, (5) trust in relation to appreciating the independent existence of the other, (6) humility indicated by a willingness to learn about and from the other, (7) hope in experiencing the richness and sense of the possible in the present, (8) courage in a sense of willingness to go into the unknown.[7]

Leininger contends that caring is one of the most critical and essential ingredients of health, human development and relatedness, well-being, and survival.[3] She saw a relationship between caring and curing: "Caring is essential to curing and pervades all efforts to help an individual recover after an illness and be cured."[8] Furthermore, Leininger believes that systematic research to describe clearly caring behavior, values, and practices in nursing is needed to incorporate that knowledge into education and practice. Her studies of cross-cultural care phenomena are in progress.

Turning to specific completed research studies on care, a few can be cited. Linn investigated the care-cure attitudes of medical and nurse faculties and their students and found that the medical faculty was more cure-oriented than were their students, and the nurse faculty was more care-oriented than the medical faculty and medical-nurse student groups.[9] No statistically significant difference was found between the means of the nursing students and that of the nursing faculty who were studied. Linn also found that medical students were more likely to place greater importance on patient cure than care. Nursing students gave more importance to care. She concluded that the findings may reflect a trend among physicians-to-be of increasing sensitivity to nonmedical factors associated with illness. This trend, together with the increasing numbers of nurses being prepared to assume more cure-oriented roles, could result in different types of health services and different professional or technical role changes. Linn qualified her conclusions by formulating the assumption that nurses in cure-oriented roles will not become unconcerned about the importance of care and emotional support. Clearly, nurses scored higher in care aspects than did the physicians in this study.[9]

Baer, Davitz, and Lieb studied inferences by nurses, social workers, and physicians in response to patients' verbal and nonverbal physical and psychologic distress.[10] Nurses in this study did not fare so well: social workers were shown to detect the greatest distress. Baer et al raised the following questions: Have nurses become so busy that they no longer perceive patients' pain? Does the social worker's response indicate greater identification with the patient? Is it because of her educational background? Is it because she is not intimately involved with the patients' physical care, or have nurses and doctors blocked their awareness of patient needs with their own needs? Furthermore, Baer et al found that all groups inferred greater pain from verbal than from nonverbal clues.[10] This tarnishes nurses' professed pride in their ability to perceive and identify patient care needs.

Wallston et al studied the effects of intervention designed to enhance the person-centeredness of nurses' responses.[11] A two-phase design was used in which nurses in Group I did not receive the intervention, which consisted of a review accompanied by illustrative examples of helpful responses, while nurses in Group II did receive the intervention. The data showed that the intervention was effective in increasing Group II's person-centeredness. This research indicated that significant improvement in judged person-centeredness could be obtained.[11]

Smolinski studied differences in perception of care between patients and nurses.[12] The problem was further subdivided into differences between patient and nurse perceptions in relation to general, physical, and psychologic needs of patients in the nursing care situation. No overall differences in these perceptions were found; however, comments made by both nurses and patients emphasized the importance of the supportive role in nursing care.[12]

In a 1975 study, Henry identified major care categories of technical, communication, and interpersonal nurse behavior that indicated how caring is perceived by patients.[13] The three major categories were: (1) what the nurse does, (2) how the nurse does it, and (3) how much the nurse does. Henry's findings revealed that 51% of subject responses were contained in the category, "how much the nurse does"; 48% of subject responses combined the categories of "what the nurse does," with "how the nurse does it."[13] Based on these data, Henry drew three overall conclusions: (1) nurses need to capitalize on nursing skill procedures by maximizing the inherent opportunity for communication, (2) patients see nursing procedures as necessary, and when the nurse performs these procedures, it indicates that she cares both for and about them, (3) patients want to know both the nurse and the person who is the nurse.[13]

Stetler investigated the listening and verbal behavior of nurses in the form of various communication techniques and vocal behaviors.[14] Nonverbal factors were not investigated in the study, which used an audio-taped simulated encounter between a nurse and a pathophysiologically ill actress-patient. Stetler assumed that verbal, nonverbal, and vocal communication are integral elements within any communication situation. She further suggested that the key to the perception of empathetic understanding lies in a complex combination of all three, with congruency among the three as the factor of primary importance. Stetler recommended that the study be enlarged to incorporate investigation of nonverbal variables; videotape provides an avenue through which this is possible.[14]

Concepts found in the review of the literature regarding caring and care include empathy, involvement, sharing, listening, honesty, person-centeredness, and verbal, nonverbal, and technical skills. These concepts are often found in the literature, and they indicate that some agreement is beginning to evolve among nurses regarding which concepts are associated with the phenomenon of caring and care.

PROBLEM AND PURPOSE OF THIS STUDY

The investigator pursued this study on the basis that research is needed to determine interpersonal relationship content in nursing. This content is primarily taught from tradition or authority, learned by imitative behavior, and practiced nonsystematically by many nurses. Through research, caring content in nursing could be taught from a scientific knowledge base, and the quality of patient care and cure should improve. The investigator also desired to pursue nursing research on care behaviors to establish care as the focus of the profession and the health care system.

The central focus of this study was to determine which verbal and nonverbal caring and uncaring nurse behaviors, and which technical competency and incompetency ones in the nurse-patient relationship were perceived as caring by female and male subjects.

Hypotheses

The study problem was addressed via 15 null hypotheses. Verbal and nonverbal caring and uncaring nurse behavior, and technical competency and incompetency nurse behavior were independent variables combined to form main effects and two-way, three-way, and four-way interaction effects. The sex of the subject, another independent variable, was an added dimension of the study problem. For purposes of this chapter, only the following null hypotheses considering the sex-of-subject perception factor relative to verbal, nonverbal, and competency nurse behavior variables are addressed in depth:

1. There is no significant difference, as noted by perceptions of female subjects and of male subjects, between verbal caring and verbal uncaring nurse behavior.

2. There is no significant difference, as noted by perceptions of female subjects and of male subjects, between nonverbal caring and nonverbal uncaring nurse behavior.

3. There is no significant difference, as noted by perceptions of female subjects and of male subjects, between verbal caring and verbal uncaring nurse behavior, whether the nurse behavior is also technically competent or technically incompetent.

4. There is no significant difference, as noted by perceptions of female subjects and of male subjects, between nonverbal caring and nonverbal uncaring nurse behavior, whether the nurse behavior is also technically competent or technically incompetent.

METHODOLOGY

Design

A 2 x 2 x 2 x 2 factorial experimental research design was used to test the simultaneous effects of the independent variables on the dependent variables. Videotape segments provided the method through which the manipulations were performed.

Subjects and Setting

An availability sample of 240 undergraduate students attending a commuter regional campus of a four-year state-supported university was selected. The regional campus is located in the North Central United States. Educational opportunities at this campus include the first two years of general education courses leading to a variety of baccalaureate degrees, 16 two-year associate degree technical programs, and occasional upper-level credit courses. The majority of students attending classes at this campus are enrolled in courses leading to an associate degree.[15,16]

Of the approximately 1000 students registered at the campus, all were eligible for inclusion in the study with the exception of those who had been enrolled in or had completed courses in nursing. The 240 subjects were divided equally between the sexes; the mean age was 22 years; and the subjects ranged in age from 17 to 45 years

The independent variables consisted of: (1) verbal caring and verbal uncaring communication, (2) nonverbal caring and nonverbal uncaring behaviors, (3) technically competent and technically incompetent nurse behaviors, and (4) sex of study subjects.

The verbal, nonverbal, and technical nurse's behaviors were displayed by a nurse interacting with a patient in a short, contrived videotape. Because material explicitly addressing the study's independent variables was not available, the eight segments were written by the investigator for the study. Content for the segments was derived from the investigator's background and from review of the literature. The basic format, identical in all segments, showed a male patient admitted to a private room on a medical-surgical service for treatment following an injury. The stimulus person was female. Persons playing the nurse and patient roles had performance experience.

The dependent variables consisted of the subjects' scores on three instruments.

Script Nursing Behaviors Used in Study

The nurse behaviors contained in the scripts were defined as follows:

1. Verbal caring was based upon use of communication techniques. The nurse provided information, shared observations about the patient's apparent emotional state, explained procedures, and validated the

patient's implied thoughts and feelings. The nurse acknowledged the patient's feelings and used reflection and selective reflection methods.[17]

2. Verbal uncaring was based upon use of communication blocks. The nurse discounted the patient's concerns, reprimanded, gave the patient advice, requested explanations, and belittled the patient's thoughts and feelings. She made judgments, used clichés, and agreed with the patient inappropriately.[17]

3. Nonverbal caring was based upon the nurse's ability to interact comfortably with the patient. She walked calmly into the patient unit and stood comfortably at the bedside. She pulled up a chair and sat down, remained seated, and rested her arm on the bed as she interacted with the patient. She exhibited an interested and attentive facial expression throughout the interaction.

4. Nonverbal uncaring was defined by the nurse's discomfort in the patient unit. The nurse frequently stood behind and leaned on a chair located at the foot of the bed, frowned, showed an impatient or tense facial expression, and often rested both hands on her hips. She sighed loudly, moved away from the bedside, checked her wristwatch, and looked away from the patient during the interaction and nursing care procedures.

5. Competent nursing behavior was based upon knowledge and technical nursing performance. The nurse counted the intravenous drop-rate per minute and calculated the approximate length of time the fluid would last, and retaped the intravenous tubing based on visual assessment. She checked the nasogastric tube for proper position without difficulty, and switched the suction machine to the "off" position based on knowledge and assessment of the patient's condition. She checked the patient's leg position in the splint, assessed its condition, and smoothly administered various nursing procedures.

6. Incompetent nursing behavior was exhibited by the nurse's overall hesitant and uncertain manner in carrying out the nursing tasks. She was unable to calculate the number of intravenous drops per minute or the approximate length of time the fluid would last, and she was unsure about the condition of the intravenous site. She frequently exhibited a puzzled facial expression, shrugged her shoulders, and did not explain procedures to the patient. She made nursing observations hesitantly and had difficulty remembering concepts underlying the nursing procedures. She held and manipulated equipment and supplies awkwardly and knocked a piece of equipment from the bedside table to the floor.

Script Pretest

Three panels of persons—professional nurses, undergraduate psychology research students, and second-year associate degree nursing students—participated in the script pretest to determine if the intended behavior combinations were in fact communicated by the scripts. Each participant read one script and responded to a three-item, investigator-developed, seven-point Likert-type questionnaire addressing the verbal, nonverbal, and competency nurse behavior levels.

Data in the form of means generated by the pretest questionnaire revealed that the scripts, as intended, did describe verbal caring and verbal uncaring communication patterns, nonverbal caring and nonverbal uncaring behaviors, and technical nursing competency and technical nursing incompetency skill levels.

Instruments

The dependent variables consisted of three instruments adapted by the investigator for use in this study. (1) The *Social Distance Scale* developed by Bogardus contains social contacts that vary in their degree of sympathetic understanding and personal-group distance.[18] (2) Kirchner's *Attitudes of Special Groups Toward the Employment of Older Persons Scale*, known as the *Attitudes Toward Employment Scale*, was adapted and used. This scale measures various attitudes of the employee in the work setting.[19] (3) The *Slater Nursing Competencies Rating Scale* developed by Wandelt and Stewart was the last scale adapted by the investigator for use in the study. Items from the Psychosocial Individual and Communication sections were chosen to be included. This scale tests various actions relative to patient care.[20] The three scales, adapted to contain 11 items each, were identified as Questionnaire #1, Questionnaire #2, and Questionnaire #3. Each item on the scales was measured by means of a seven-point Likert-type method. Values of one to seven were assigned to the responses as follows: 1—strongly agree, 2—agree, 3—somewhat agree, 4—neutral, 5—somewhat disagree, 6—disagree, and 7—strongly disagree. The range of the total score per instrument was 11 to 77.

Data Collection

Data was collected during two consecutive semesters in 1980. The videotaped segments were randomly assigned for viewing by the subject groups, each containing 15 females and 15 males by the Random Permutation Table. A signed consent form was requested from each subject. For purposes of control, all subjects were presented with an audiotaped introduction and participation instructions, after which subject signatures were obtained on the consent forms. The videotaped segment was then shown. Questionnaires #1 and #2 were administered. Questionnaire #3 was addressed last because it spoke directly to and evaluated the various nurse behaviors displayed in the scripts.

ANALYSIS OF DATA

Descriptive statistical measures were used to report the subject demographic data. Postinvestigation alpha reliability coefficient levels were determined for the investigator-adapted dependent variables. Means were computed on all independent variable data. Four-way analysis of variance procedures were used to test significant main and interaction effects exerted on the dependent variables by the independent variables. The preset $p < 0.05$ level of statistically significant difference, based on the F test result, was used as the criterion for rejection of the hypotheses.

SUMMARY OF FINDINGS

Overall, the findings resulted in identified independently important differences between and among the variables of verbal and nonverbal nurse behavior and level of technical competency when predicting preference for nurse behavior. Congruence between and among the behavior variables was a significant factor in relationship to perceived nurse behavior. When the nurse in the script portrayed verbal caring, nonverbal caring, and technical competency behavior, both females and males exhibited a definite preference for her behavior. Furthermore, when the nurse in the script portrayed verbal uncaring, nonverbal uncaring, and technical incompetency behavior, both females and males indicated that they rejected her behavior.

Even though the variables of verbal and nonverbal nurse behavior and technical level of competency were not judged to be statistically different as main effects in relation to sex-of-subject differences, these behaviors were statistically significantly different when tested as interaction effects. In general, males tended to use the nurse's level of technical skill performance as a criterion for judging nurses' behavior, while females tended to use the nurse's interpersonal awareness behavior.

Additional Findings

Determination of postinvestigation alpha reliability coefficient levels was performed on the investigator-adapted dependent variable scales. The alpha levels for each scale remained high, which indicated that the adaptation process in use prior to this study did not alter the scales' levels of internal consistency. Figure 12–1 compares the original reliability levels for each scale with the reliability levels obtained after adaptation and use in this study.[20,21]

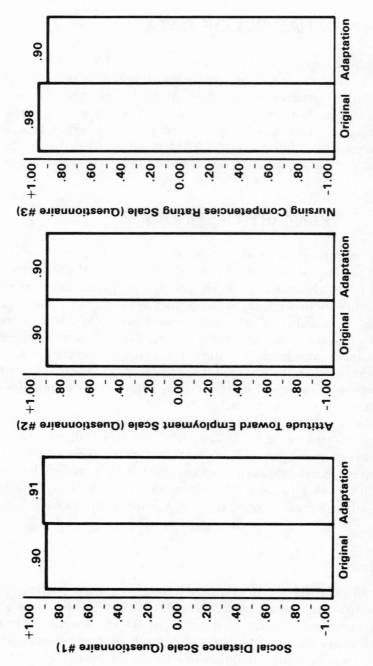

Figure 12-1. Original scale reliability levels and reliability levels after adaptation and use in study. (Reprinted by permission of J. Gerontol 12:2, 1957; Wandelt A, Stewart DS: Slater Nursing Competencies Rating Scale. New York, Appleton-Century-Crofts, 1975; and Bogardus ES: Sociol Soc Research 17:265, 1933.)

DISCUSSION OF FINDINGS

Because the study identified gender-related effects relative to preference for nurses' behavior, the hypotheses involving statistically significant sex-of-subject interactions are discussed in depth according to the data generated by the three dependent variable scales: social attractiveness, job effectiveness, and interpersonal awareness. Specifically, the female-male effect in the present study reflected even slightly different results in relationship to judging nurses' behavior in terms of social attractiveness, overall level of work effectiveness, and degree of interpersonal relationship skill.

Social Attractiveness

In addressing the nurse's behavior relative to social attractiveness, the sex-of-the subject variable interacted significantly at the two-way and three-way interaction effect levels with the verbal and technical competency variables.

Regarding the two-way interaction effect level, the data showed that the verbal caring nurse was found to be significantly more attractive to the female subjects, as indicated by the lower mean score. Furthermore, there was rejection by the female subjects of the verbal uncaring nurse behavior, as indicated by the highest mean score. Verbal caring behavior was better liked by females, and at the same time, verbal uncaring behavior was significantly rejected by females. Males did not judge this difference so greatly as did the females. Table 12–1 displays these data.

Table 12-1. Mean Difference between Verbal Nurse Behavior vs Sex-of-Subject Scores

Treatment						
Verbal Caring		**Verbal Uncaring**				
Female Subjects X	Male Subjects X	Female Subjects X	Male Subjects X	df	F	p
43.03	46.00	52.33	48.68	1/224	4.947	.027

$n = 240$.

At the three-way interaction effect level of verbal vs competency vs sex-of-subject variables, females and males reported preference for verbal caring, technically competent nurse behavior as based on the low mean scores for the nurse who portrayed these behaviors. There was highly significant rejection, again by the females, for the nurse displaying verbal uncaring, technically incompetent behaviors. These data indicate that verbal caring behavior acted as an overriding effect for the females, in that even though the nurse was technically incompetent, she remained attractive if she showed verbal caring behavior. At the same time, the males indicated preference for the verbal uncaring, technically competent nurse. Table 12–2 summarizes these data.

Table 12-2. Mean Difference between Verbal vs Competency Nurse Behavior vs Sex-of-Subject Scores

| Verbal Caring | | | | Verbal Uncaring | | | | | | |
| Technical Competence | | Technical Incompetence | | Technical Competence | | Technical Incompetence | | | | |
Female Subjects X	Male Subjects X	Female Subjects X	Male Subjects X	Female Subjects X	Male Subjects X	Female Subjects X	Male Subjects X	df	F	p
40.90	40.87	45.17	51.13	48.43	47.73	56.23	49.63	1/224	4.000	.047

n = 240.

Table 12-3. Mean Difference between Verbal Nurse Behavior vs Sex-of-Subject Scores

| Verbal Caring | | Verbal Uncaring | | | | |
Female Subjects X	Male Subjects X	Female Subjects X	Male Subjects X	df	F	p
50.38	51.90	61.33	57.62	1/224	4.281	.040

Treatment

$n = 240$.

Job Effectiveness

In judging the nurse's behavior in relation to overall level of work capability, the sex-of-subject variable interacted significantly at the two-way and three-way interaction levels, this time with both verbal and nonverbal behavior variables as well as with the technical competency variable. Again, females tended to be more attuned to verbal and nonverbal behavior, while males based the nurse's level of work capability and job effectiveness on degree of technical competency.

Specifically regarding the verbal variable vs sex-of-subject variable at the two-way interaction level, the data showed that the verbal caring nurse was perceived to be more job-effective by both the female subjects and the male subjects as indicated by the lowest mean scores. Furthermore, these findings indicated rejection, again by the female subjects, as noted by the highest mean score. The male subjects indicated more acceptance of the verbal uncaring nurse behavior than did the females. Additionally, males showed rejection of the verbal uncaring nurse behavior, but to a lesser degree than did the females. Table 12-3 contains the verbal vs sex-of-subject data. When examining the nonverbal vs sex-of-subject two-way interaction effect, the same overall result is evidenced. Table 12-4 portrays these data.

Table 12-4. Mean Difference between Nonverbal Nurse Behavior vs Sex-of-Subject Scores

| Nonverbal Caring | | Nonverbal Uncaring | | | | |
Female Subjects X	Male Subjects X	Female Subjects X	Male Subjects X	df	F	p
49.95	53.23	61.77	56.28	1/224	12.012	.001

Treatment

$n = 240$.

Upon examination of the three-way interaction effect of nonverbal vs competency vs sex-of-subject variables, the data showed that females perceived the nurse who displayed nonverbal caring, technically competent behavior to be more job-effective and competent in relationship to employment. This effect was based on the low mean score for the nurse who exhibited these behaviors. Furthermore, there was rejection by both sexes of the nurse who displayed nonverbal uncaring, technically incompetent behavior, as evidenced by the highest mean scores. Additionally, there was a significant female-male effect in terms of caring vs competency nurse behaviors. Females rated the nurse who portrayed nonverbal uncaring, technically competent nurse behavior as less attractive in relationship to work effectiveness and capability than the males. Relative to work capability behavior combinations, males preferred nonverbal uncaring, technically competent nurse behavior over the nonverbal caring, technically incompetent nurse behavior preferred by females. Table 12–5 presents these data.

Interpersonal Awareness

In relationship to measuring the nurse's degree of interpersonal awareness ability, the sex-of-subject variable interacted significantly at the two-way and three-way effect levels with the nonverbal behavior and technical competency variables. The data reported that the variables of nonverbal nurse behavior and technical level of competency are important to both females and males. Females, however, are more sensitive to nonverbal behavior than males and tended to judge the nurse's ability for interpersonal relationships on the degree of nonverbal caring. Males, again, are less sensitive to the nonverbal behavior and tended to judge the nurse's behavior on the degree of technical competency.

Specifically, in relation to the two-way nonverbal vs sex-of-subject interaction effect, the data indicated, by the lowest mean score, that the nurse who showed nonverbal caring behavior was perceived by the females to be more interpersonally sensitive to, interested in, and concerned for the patient. Furthermore, nonverbal caring nurse behavior was preferred significantly over nonverbal uncaring behavior by females, resulting in a female rejection effect. Females were more sensitive to nonverbal caring behavior than males; however, both groups responded positively to the nonverbal caring behavior pattern. Overall, males responded positively to nonverbal caring nurse behavior and negatively to nonverbal uncaring behavior, but not so forcefully as did the females. Table 12–6 displays these data.

Relative to the three-way interaction effect of nonverbal vs competency vs sex-of-subject variables, the data showed, according to the lowest mean score, that females found nonverbal caring, technically competent nurse behavior more interpersonally sensitive and effective. Furthermore, there was highly significant rejection, by the females as well as the males, for the nurse who displayed nonverbal uncaring, technically incompetent behavior. This rejection effect is evidenced by the highest mean scores. Female subjects rejected the

Table 12-5. Mean Difference between Nonverbal vs Competency Nurse Behavior vs Sex-of-Subject Scores

Nonverbal Caring				Nonverbal Uncaring						
Technical Competence		Technical Incompetence		Technical Competence		Technical Incompetence				
Female Subjects X	Male Subjects X	Female Subjects X	Male Subjects X	Female Subjects X	Male Subjects X	Female Subjects X	Male Subjects X	df	F	p
42.37	46.90	57.53	59.57	60.10	50.40	63.43	62.17	1/224	4.671	.032

n = 240.

nonverbal uncaring, technically competent nurse behavior to a greater degree, however, than did the males. In general, the data suggested that females reacted to the degree of nonverbal caring or uncaring behavior, while males appeared to react to the degree of technical competency or incompetency. Table 12–7 summarizes these data.

Table 12-6. Mean Difference between Nonverbal Nurse Behavior vs Sex-of-Subject Scores

Treatment						
Nonverbal Caring		Nonverbal Uncaring				
Female Subjects X	Male Subjects X	Female Subjects X	Male Subjects X	df	F	p
46.95	50.38	61.63	58.03	1/224	8.229	.005

$n = 240$.

These findings showed a trend throughout the study for females to react repeatedly to verbal and/or nonverbal nurse behavior in terms of making judgments about the nurse, while males repeatedly reacted to technical skill level relative to these judgments. Verbal and nonverbal caring and technical competency nurse behavior, according to this study, occupy positions of substantive importance regarding an individual's preference for nurse behavior.

CONCLUSIONS AND IMPLICATIONS FOR NURSES AND NURSING

1. Persons value verbal, nonverbal, and technical nurse behavior. Exhibiting verbal and nonverbal caring and exercising technically competent behavior are important as nurses interact with and care for patients; congruence among the behaviors is an added important factor.

   Nurse educators should continue to teach verbal, nonverbal, and technical skills, allowing equal time for the three areas. Verbal and nonverbal learning opportunities could be pointed out to a greater degree in conjunction with the technical competency, task learning opportunities, for it is impossible to separate totally the three behavior areas.

   Choice of nursing instructor for the verbal and nonverbal interactive skill areas may be important. An individual who is comfortable with the less structured, person-centered, and personally interactive format might more effectively occupy this position.

Table 12-7. Mean Difference between Nonverbal vs Competency Nurse Behavior vs Sex-of-Subject Scores

		Treatment									
Nonverbal Caring				Nonverbal Uncaring							
Technical Competence		Technical Incompetence		Technical Competence		Technical Incompetence					
Female Subjects X	Male Subjects X	Female Subjects X	Male Subjects X	Female Subjects X	Male Subjects X	Female Subjects X	Male Subjects X	*df*	*F*	*p*
38.57	44.20	55.33	56.57	60.13	53.03	63.13	63.03	1/224	5.405	.032

n = 240.

Additional continuing education and in-service minicourses which focus on verbal and nonverbal content, skills, and practice could be offered so that nurses who have been involved in the work force and who may not have been rewarded for these behaviors can update their interpersonal skills. These educational/service opportunities could also assist the nurse returning to active employment.

Tools presently used to measure nursing care outcomes tend to look in greater depth at technical competency nurse behavior. This is in direct disagreement with the findings of the present study, which focus attention on the need for verbal and nonverbal nurse behavior in addition to technical competency.

Regarding cost, a dollar value has not been assigned to nursing care behavior in general, much less to the verbal and nonverbal nurse behavior that represents an important area of nursing practice, according to the results of this study. This may represent a basic consideration in job satisfaction and may be a prime factor in the attempt to advance nursing to the level of a recognized health service profession.

2. Persons have different preferences for nurse behavior. Some of the preferences may be based on gender. Therefore, it is important for nurses to display verbal and nonverbal caring behavior as well as technical competency when caring for both female and male patients, even though males overly react to the competency behavior and females overly react to the interactive verbal and nonverbal nurse behavior.

Nursing education processes may be affected by the female-male effect evidenced in these study results. Female nursing instructors may evaluate their male students, not only in relation to technical skill competency levels, but also in relation to the instructor's own verbal and nonverbal nurse behavior values. The converse may also be true: male nursing faculty may place less value on the verbal and nonverbal nurse behavior that their female students tend to stress and value.

If the individuals in charge of nursing, namely the male-dominated group of physicians and administrators, tend to value the technical competency component of nursing, as these study results indicate, nurse educators may have to counsel prospective students about the realities of the nursing practice reward system: If the prospective student is male, the rewards for technical competency are available. If the prospective student is female, she should be made aware of the gender-related behavior values. The female student can then be prepared to accept reality, prepared to handle the disappointments that are likely to occur relative to her values and needs, and assisted to learn methods and behaviors that will help her cope with reality and take steps to change it.

The female-male effect evident throughout this study — in relationship to the male tendency to place greater emphasis on the technical skill competency level when judging nurse behavior — may be due in part to the growth and development and socialization processes directed at males in our society. Males are socialized to be less emotional, less subjective, and more objective in their thinking processes, attitudes, and behavior than are females. Therefore, it is hypothesized that males may have been unable to respond overtly on paper to the verbal and nonverbal caring behaviors exhibited by the nurse.

The opposite may be true for females: Growth and development and socialization processes of females in our society allow them to be more emotional, more subjective, and less objective in their thinking processes, attitudes, and behavior than males. Again, it can be hypothesized that the females may have been unable to separate critically the feeling behavior from the technical task component in evaluating the nurse's behavior.

Informal nurse peer evaluation may be affected by the female-male effect. A male nurse, while personally judging a female nurse colleague's behavior, will tend to use the technical competency value as the judgment criterion, based on the study results. The female nurse colleague is likely to place her value emphasis on the verbal and nonverbal behavior aspects.

The opposite may be true for the reverse peer couple: The female nurse judging a male nurse colleague in relation to professional behavior will tend to judge the male nurse's behavior on the basis of the verbal and nonverbal behavior she values. He, however, is likely to be concerned to a greater degree with technical competency.

Formal supervisor nurse evaluation processes may be affected by the female-male effect in much the same ways as just described regarding the informal peer evaluation activity. More serious consequences may occur in relation to this evaluation because pay rewards and promotion opportunities may be placed in jeopardy by the differences in the female-male nurse-behavior value system.

The gender effect identified by this study may represent one of the reasons women are leaving nursing practice. If women have entered nursing in order to practice the verbal and nonverbal caring behaviors they value along with technical skills, they probably have not been rewarded for performing the interactive behaviors. When they find that they are unable to cope with the sex-based behavior preference differences, they may choose other areas of employment.

Since the health care delivery system is administered to a large extent by male physicians and administrative persons, it follows that the male value of technical competency will be reflected in the policies of the agency. This value is likely, therefore, to be in evidence in the reward system.

RECOMMENDATIONS FOR RESEARCH

This study should be replicated in other parts of the country using different subject groups. Groups to sample could include older people, nurses, non-nurses, physicians, health care agency administrators, people who have been hospitalized, and those who have not been hospitalized. Additional studies could be carried out in relation to nursing evaluation tools to include or increase the amount of verbal and nonverbal nurse behavior. Further research could be done relative to nursing care outcome measurements in terms of adding or increasing the verbal and nonverbal behavior factors. An exploration of technical competency and verbal and nonverbal caring behavior in the nurse-patient relationship relative to cost should be conducted.

REFERENCES

1. Harlem OK: Care has lagged behind cure: research in nursing needed to create a proper balance. Nordisk Medicin 93:69, 1978.
2. Ray MA: A philosophical analysis of caring within nursing. In Leininger M(ed): Caring: An Essential Human Need. Thorofare, NJ, Charles B. Slack, Inc., 1981.
3. Leininger M: The phenomenon of caring: importance, research questions and theoretical considerations. In Leininger M(ed): Caring: An Essential Human Need. Thorofare, NJ, Charles B. Slack, Inc., 1981.
4. Leininger M: Caring: An Essential Human Need. Thorofare, NJ, Charles B. Slack, Inc., 1981.
5. Goldsborough J: Involvement. Nursing 69:66-68, 1969.
6. Velazquez JM: Alienation. Nursing 69:301–304, 1969.
7. Mayeroff M: On Caring. New York, Perennial Library, Harper & Row Publications, 1971.
8. Leininger M: Caring: a central focus of nursing and health care services. Nursing and Health Care 1:135–176, 1980.
9. Linn LS: A survey of the "care-cure" attitudes of physicians, nurses, and their students. Nursing Forum 14:145–159, 1975.
10. Baer E, Davitz LJ, Lieb R: Inferences of physical pain and psychological distress. Nursing Research 19:388–392, 1970.
11. Wallston KA, Cohen BD, Wallston BS, et al: Increasing nurses' person-centeredness. Nursing Research 17:156–159, 1978.
12. Smolinski LM: Patient perception of care received and nurse perception of care given regarding the same nursing acts. Unpublished doctoral dissertation, The Catholic University of America, 1975.
13. Henry OM: Nurse behaviors perceived by patients as indicators of caring. Unpublished doctoral dissertation, The Catholic University of America, 1975.
14. Stetler CB: Relationship of perceived empathy to nurses' communication. Nursing Research 26:432–438, 1977.
15. Regional Campuses Annual Report. Kent, Ohio, Kent State University, 1977–1978.
16. Regional Campuses Annual Report. Kent, Ohio, Kent State University, 1980–1981.
17. Nurse-Patient Interaction. Costa Mesa, CA, Concept Media, 1970.
18. Bogardus ES: A social distance scale. Sociol Social Research 17:265–271, 1933.

19. Kirchner WK: The attitudes of special groups toward the employment of older persons. J Gerontol 12:216–220, 1957.
20. Wandelt MA, Stewart DS: Slater Nursing Competencies Rating Scale. New York, Appleton-Century-Crofts, 1975.
21. Shaw ME, Wright JM: Scales for the Measurement of Attitudes. New York, McGraw-Hill Book Company, 1967.

13

Compadrazgo: A Caring Phenomenon Among Urban Latinos and Its Relationship to Health

An important and long overdue area of study is that of human caring. Considering that this function may be central to the continuance of the human species on earth, it is remarkable that so little attention, except in the case of early child development, has been paid to those human impulses and behaviors that nurture, assist, guide, and protect. Under the leadership of Leininger, important strides have been made in the research on caring that reflect both quantitative and qualitative perspectives of research methods.[1,2] Both types will help determine to what extent caring behaviors make a difference in nursing, especially since caring has been cogently argued to be nursing's central focus.[3]

This chapter examines a form of social alliance, *compadrazgo*, that has for centuries until the present day been deeply imbedded in the Latino culture. It demonstrates what implications such a system may have for nursing's caring activities when viewed from a broad sociocultural perspective.

COMPADRAZGO AS A FORM OF UNIVERSAL SOCIAL ALLIANCE

Social bonds have been forged since earliest human history, and in very early times they were undoubtedly formed among those individuals in close proximity, namely kin. As Robin Fox points out, kinship systems have to do with early man's attempts to deal with the "basic facts of life—mating, gestation, parenthood, socialization, siblingship, etc." and further, "part of (man's) enormous success in the evolutionary struggle lies in his ability to manipulate these relationships to advantage . . . in order to survive, and beyond survival, to prosper."[4]

Social alliances are formed both within kinship systems and outside them. They are, essentially, maneuvers to extend social bonds beyond biologic realms and to enter into agreements of mutual interdependence and reciprocity that hold promise of additional security or advantage.[5] There are numerous social alliances that have been and continue to be interwoven in social intercourse. Levi-Strauss argues that in traditional societies, formerly termed "primitive," basic kinship groups are part of a fluidly operating system of alliances that are made via marriage, so that moving women around within a system or within several overlapping systems provides for far-reaching and complex ties. These ties reflect obligations and responsibilities to assist in case of an enemy attack, to use kin territories, or to employ other prerogatives.[6]

In recent times, the "old school tie" network is well known as a method of climbing corporate or academic ladders. It is a type of "brotherhood" whereby proteges are anointed and given open doors that are not readily available to those not selected. Benefits are not readily available to those not selected. The benefits are intended to be mutual and can extend over a broad spectrum, ie, economic, social, political, and emotional areas.

Compadrazgo is more nearly comparable with the traditional, as opposed to the modern-industrial, versions of social alliance, since it involves family-type links and not primarily market or workplace unions. It is a form of alliance that traces its roots back to feudal European days, with flexible attributes and persistence over time.[7] Embedded in the social matrix of Latinos, *compadrazgo* can be identified as follows:

1. It is a fictive kin tie, ie, it is not biologically or legally ascribed, as in the case of blood relations or marital alliances. Once entered into, however, it assumes various dimensions of affect and responsibility similar to other familiar bonds of filiality.

2. It has a ritualistic aspect, ie, the relationship between the parties is initiated most often via a religious blessing, whether the occasion be, for example, the baptism of an infant, or the blessing of a house.

3. It is coparenthood—as opposed to *padrinazgo*, which is godparenthood— with the emphasis on the relationship that is established between parent and sponsor; these individuals call one another *compadre*, both as a form of address and in future reference to one another.[8]

COMPADRAZGO AS A TYPE OF CARING

The title *compadre*, or *comadre* in the case of women, is imbued with great warm feeling and deep respect as the central, pervading attribute of the relationship. In the author's own research, primarily among people of Mexican heritage living in a northern United States urban area, descriptions of the relationship have been as follows: "It's like having a grandmother, aunt, sister, mother all wrapped up in one," "this is something that is so deep it goes to the soul," "it's hard to describe it because it's something deeply felt," and "nothing can destroy it because it grows and goes deeper all the time." It has also been described as "you might be close to your brother but not like this; with your brother you have fights or bad times, with your *compadre* it is only good—respect, honor—good things always."[9] Apparently, when functioning ideally, this may be a type of brotherly love without sibling rivalry. It is of interest to note that this is a caring, supportive relationship that involves men as well as women. The warmth is expressed most often about relationships of *comadre* with *comadre*, and *compadre* with *compadre*, but this does not make the male or female pairing mutually exclusive, for there are references by women to their *compadres*, and vice versa. Expressions of deep respect, and what can most nearly be described as loving expressions of satisfaction with the relationship, are nearly always present.

Compadrazgo is clearly a caring phenomenon, embedded in a rich fabric of sociocultural practice that is universal in nature. It reflects nearly all the components identified by Leininger as principles of caring phenomena; most specifically, it is a culturally embedded process related to specific social structural features—humanistically oriented, therapeutically linked, and with symbolic referents.[10]

The caring in these relationships is conscious and explicit, an alliance that includes a close, socially sanctioned agreement of future mutual reciprocity. Sometimes the caring is expressed by gift-giving and by special hospitality. There are also occasions when economic aid is offered or requested. At times, the important aspect of the alliance is the status that accrues from having a close involvement with a person who holds a place of special importance in the community. One of the key aspects of the relationship, however, appears to be alleviating concerns about the future; that is, in case one should need assistance of some sort, either economic or emotional, one has a bank of resources upon which he knows he may draw should the need arise. At the same time, he is ready to be called on in turn by his *compadre* in a similar manner.

There is a discernible feeling of ready generosity that is expressed when the topic of *compadres* is mentioned. For example, one woman with whom the author talked said that when she became ill shortly after the birth of her first baby, her *comadre* took the infant to her own home and cared for him, while coming in at regular intervals to cook, clean, and nurse the ailing woman. Another woman told the author that when she needed a ride, "I could always ask my *comadre*—and she helped me every day," an arrangement that went on for weeks. A man who was unemployed talked about managing to get along "because I have my family." In talking further, it became apparent that intermingled with the designation "family" were several very involved *compadres*.

CARING AS A COPING STRATEGY
WITH RESPECT TO ILLNESS

Is caring, such as we see in the social form of *compadrazgo,* a coping device that ameliorates some of the stress of daily living? Empirically, the answer would be "yes." When functioning ideally, both its expressive and instrumental aspects, as well as the insurance it promises relative to future needs, give the process an almost wholly positive cast. One exception to the primarily positive assessments of *compadrazgo* is the presence of usually unexpressed ambivalence that participants in the system may feel about the demands upon them to stifle negative feelings toward their specially designated "relations."[11] In the author's research among an urban population, it was reported that where *compadrazgo* is not functioning well—for example, when *compadres* are selected from among friends or relatives of one spouse and are not compatible with the other spouse—the relationship is simply not activated. Put another way, it is left "to die on the vine." While there can be no positive outcome in such a situation, neither, it appears, is there one of a negative nature.

In terms of methodologic definition, which would make the concept amenable to research on coping strategies, *compadrazgo* can be readily assigned to the category of "social resources" (in the parlance of social research). This research grouping includes family, friends, neighbors, coworkers, and persons within community fraternal organizations, all of whom are potentially able to be drawn upon as part of a given individual's repertoire of coping strategies.[12]

Cobb has defined social support as information leading an individual to believe "that he is cared for and loved, esteemed, and a member of a network of mutual obligations."[13] Cobb and others, with some reservations, take the position that generally social supports are protective with respect to illness, regardless of whether the illness is predominantly physiologic or emotional.[13,14] Furthermore, "the sheer richness and variety of responses and resources that one can bring to bear in coping with life-strains may be more important in shielding one's self from emotional stress than the nature and content of any single coping element."[12]

Physical illnesses, especially those of a chronic, degenerative nature such as cardiovascular disorders, cancer, and pulmonary diseases, have been hypothesized as correlating with increased stresses of daily living in industrial societies. The issue is complex, however, for many other factors of modern living—such as dietary excess, substance abuse, lack of exercise, and environmentally polluting influences, not to mention genetic predisposition—are also implicated. It is important to examine those components of daily living that may be associated with illness and to discover, if possible, the coping strategies that may ameliorate their impact. Multifactorial studies that take into account genetic, environmental, sociocultural, and behavioral variables in the research model offer the greatest promise for improved understanding of these complex, intertwined issues. Methodologic problems are far from resolved with such an approach, however, and must be painstakingly addressed and acknowledged, study by study.[15]

HEALTH AND SOCIAL SUPPORTS AMONG URBAN LATINOS

A survey questionnaire was developed to tap a mixture of variables, ie, sociobiologic, economic, acculturative, stress, and social support resources, in relation to reported chronic diseases among some Latinos* living in a northern US urban area. This was an exploratory phase of research designed to ascertain which contributors to illness, if any, might subsequently be examined with greater specificity.

Method

Data were collected over a period of one year in a neighborhood that had the largest concentration of Latinos in the metropolitan area of a large northern US city. The 1980 Census records 28,970 persons of "Spanish origin" in the metropolitan area where the study was conducted, out of a total population count of 1,203,339 persons. The participant-observation method was employed in a neighborhood health center; in homes, markets, restaurants, grocery stores, churches, and parks; and at religious and nonsectarian gatherings. Informal interviews and the formal structured survey questionnaire were also data collection instruments.

Respondents were from two settings: a full-service Health and Social Services Center, and a Roman Catholic parish, both located in the urban area where a large Latino population resided. The study group, all volunteers, numbered 30 adults: 27 women and 3 men. Fifteen participated in the *compadrazgo* system, and 15 did not. Eight people spoke Spanish only and were interviewed by one of three Spanish-speaking interviewers coached by the author. The majority of the interviews were conducted in the respondents' homes.

The survey questionnaire, prepared in both English and Spanish, was designed to tap variables in the following categories:

1. *Demobiologic:* gender, age, marital status, head-of-household designation, personal and family chronic illness history (illnesses queried: diabetes, high blood pressure, chronic obstructive pulmonary disease, depression, anxiety, heart trouble, stroke, cancer, obesity).

2. *Economic Status:* residence location and mobility, income level, number of income-producing jobs, number in household.

---

*Latino designation means any person of Western Hemisphere Spanish background.

3. *Acculturation Level:* country of birth, rural or urban upbringing, length of residence in US and in urban area of current residence, citizenship status, educational attainment, occupation: current and usual, therapeutic preference when ill, use of Spanish and English media, language preference and use.

4. *Stress:* perceived—in marital, familial, household economic, occupational, and social/relational situations; significant life events; *anxiety— state* and trait.[16]

5. *Social Support Resources:* preference for and frequency of use in times of need—family, Spanish friend/neighbor, Anglo friend/neighbor, *comadre/compadre,* other persons; participation in and frequency of use— community groups such as unions, clubs, informal drinking groups; religious participation in *compadrazgo*—frequency of contact and geographic and emotional closeness.

The data were prepared for computer analysis, and the multiple regression analyses are reported here.*

Results

The multiple regression technique was employed to ascertain any overall dependence of personal chronic illness on variables when taken in the aggregate. Acculturation variables were insignificant throughout in accounting for variance in the dependent variable, Personal Chronic Illness, and so were dropped from analysis. Table 13-1 displays the variables and the order in which they entered the regression.† Family Chronic Illness History emerges as the strongest independent variable, accounting for a full 44% of variance in the dependent variable, Personal Chronic Illness ($p<.001$). Income appears next, with a negative loading, so that it is low income that explains an additional 15% of variance ($p<.01$), followed by Number in Household. Again, this is in a negative direction, indicating that there are fewer persons in the households of respondents who had more personal chronic illnesses; explained variance was 9% ($p<.05$). Stress accounted for 7% of variance in personal chronic illness ($p<.01$), and Head-of-Household Status is next at 5% explained variance ($p<.01$). The remaining two variables, Age and Social Supports, prove to be negligible in explaining variance in personal chronic illness.

*Statistical tests were performed using the system of computer programs described in Nie et al, 1975.[17]

†Used as a descriptive tool to evaluate the overall dependence of Depression on other variables. Standard regression method was employed where the order in which variables are to enter the regression is not specified, but they enter depending upon which variable explains the greatest amount of variance in the dependent variable entering first. Then the variable explaining the greatest amount of variance in conjunction with the first will enter second, and so on.[17]

Table 13-1. Summary Regression of Personal Chronic Illness on Sociobiologic, Economic, Stress, and Social Support Variables

Variables	Multiple R (cumulative)	R_2 (cum)	R_2 Change	Direction of Relationship	F
Family Chronic Illness History	.6667	.4445	— (44%)	Positive: more family chronic illness history, more personal chronic illness	p<.001
Income	.7698	.5926	.1481 (15%)	Negative: lower income, more personal chronic illness	p<.01
Number in Household	.8235	.6782	.0856 (9%)	Neg: fewer in household, more personal chronic illness	p<.05
Stress	.8672	.7520	.0738 (7%)	Pos: more stress, more personal chronic illness	p<.01
Head-of-Household Status	.8976	.8057	.0537 (5%)	Pos: head-of-household, more personal chronic illness	p<.01
Age	.9105	.8290	.0233 (2%)	Pos: higher age, more personal chronic illness	n.s.
Social Supports	.9168	.8406	.0116 (0%)	Pos: more social supports, more personal chronic illness	n.s.

n=30. Total: 84% variance in personal chronic illness explained by these variables.

Since the variable Social Supports, which included *compadre* support, showed no relationship to personal chronic illness, a regression was performed on the dependent variable, entering Stress, Social Supports, and a new variable, Having (or not Having) *Compadres,* to see what could be learned. Table 13-2 displays this regression. It can be seen that here Stress emerges with the most explanatory power among these variables, with 30% explained variance (p<.001) on the dependent variable, Personal Chronic Illness; Having *Compadres* precedes Social Supports, adding another 5% of variance explained, although this is statistically not significant.

Discussion

This survey, exploratory in nature, was undertaken to ascertain which variables from a broad array, ie, demobiologic, economic, acculturative, stress, and social support resources, might be related to chronic illness. More

**Table 13-2. Summary Regression of Personal Chronic Illness on Stress, Having
Compadres, and Social Support Variables**

Variables	Multiple R (cumulative)	R_2 (cum)	R_2 Change	Direction of Relationship	F
Stress	.5487	.3011	— (30%)	Positive: more stress, more personal chronic illness	p<.001
Has *Compadres*	.5931	.3518	.0507 (5%)	Negative: has *compadres*, less personal chronic illness	n.s.
Social Supports	.5948	.3538	.0020 (0%)	Pos: more social supports, more personal chronic illness	n.s.

n=30. Total: 35% variance in personal chronic illness explained by these variables.

important, however, it is the interplay among variables from all the categories that bears examination.

Family chronic illness history emerges as the most significant variable in predicting personal chronic illness, with 44% of variance explained by this single variable. No other variable examined comes close to this in explaining the variance in personal chronic illness. Income, at 15% of explained variance, has something to contribute when we note that it is lower income that is related to more personal chronic illness. This is in a direction that would be expected, for if family chronic illness history is potentially so determining of personal chronic illness, it may be that people with such vulnerability are less likely to have the good health and vitality, even at early ages, necessary to become high-income achievers. Conceivably, such a pattern could go back several generations. The same issue may be operating with size of household (9% of explained variance, p<.05), from which it can be seen that small households are associated with more personal chronic illness. People with one or more of the serious disorders queried in this study might be less likely to have large families, whether due to physiologic unfitness, social withdrawal during active mating years, or either poor health or low finances, which makes it less feasible to maintain a large household. On the other hand, a causal chain may be operating in the other direction, with low income exacerbating the underlying vulnerability to chronic illness, either by way of poorer subsistence opportunities or illness-inducing work conditions.

With 7% explanatory power for the Stress category relative to explained variance in chronic illness, caution must be exercised in attaching too much importance to this variable. Head-of-household status follows stress in the regression at 5% explained variance; it is possible that that role is one of potential stress untapped by the questions asked about the latter. If so, it would raise the stress factor to 12%. This is pure speculation, however, and must await more rigorous study.

The small amount of variance explained by Age is not surprising. While chronic illness is ordinarily associated with older age, this was a relatively young group (mean = 34.7 years, with a range of 20 to 67 years), so that the findings are in a direction to be expected. What is surprising (and requires further study) is the presence of so much personal chronic illness in the group as a whole (mean = 1.4 illnesses, with a low of no illnesses to a high of 5 illnesses). It should be remembered that the illnesses queried were severe and chronic in nature.

It can be seen from the data that social support resources, as tapped by this study, play a diminished role in whatever variance in personal chronic illness there is left to be explained after chronic illness family history and economic and stress variables have been counted. What this study did show is that participation in the cultural caring practice of *compadrazgo* is more meaningfully related to less personal chronic illness (5% explained variance) than the summation of all other personal and community social support resources investigated (0% explained variance). It must be noted, however, that it is not clear what part *compadrazgo* plays in relation to chronic illness. It may be that it has supportive components that minimize vulnerability to illness, or it may be that personal chronic illness has such a debilitating impact on affected individuals that they do not readily participate in extended fictive ties, or, because of their conditions, do not attract to themselves people who are capable of engaging in such relationships.

Given the fact that medical researchers have for some time maintained that a strong connection exists between disease and biologic/familial antecedents, the findings of this exploratory phase of study should not be surprising. Yet, in some ways they are. In social science research, we are used to looking at variables and findings that exclude biologic or genetic data, and in a sense, this approach permits the demographic and sociocultural relationships that are found in studies of health and illness to appear stronger than they in fact may be. Medical researchers, on the other hand, appear to omit from examination in their studies the impact that sociocultural factors may have on illness. This is to be regretted if one accepts the argument that whatever variance is accounted for by the "soft" sociocultural variables, small though it may be, should be addressed because even small percentages may tip the balance in favor of improved health.

It seems clear that a multivariant approach in studies of health that links biologic, environmental, demographic, and sociocultural factors is indeed warranted. The task of adequately operationalizing variables for reliable study, especially in the sociocultural domain, continues to be a pressing problem, however.

CONCLUSIONS

There can be little argument with the premises that guide research on caring: Caring is culturally derived; it has attributes and processes that can be transmitted (both verbal and nonverbal); and it is humanistic in its expression and function.[18] The knotty issue to be confronted, however, is how to operationalize the study of caring. The question could be asked, "Does caring make a difference in the well-being of people?" To answer that, the question of measurement must be addressed.

This chapter reports a preliminary examination of a form of caring, *compadrazgo,* which has endured in a highly flexible, dynamic form for centuries. Empirically, it appears to be a social form that has considerable supportive features in its practice. Since supportive features of social relationships have been identified as mediators between the stresses of daily life and illness in vulnerable individuals, *compadrazgo* was examined in this study to see what relationship existed between its practice and the presence of chronic illness. The findings indicate that there is a discernible relationship between personal chronic illness reported by those practicing this social form and that reported by those who do not, with those practicing it reporting fewer illnesses. The question of whether *compadrazgo* acts as a mediating influence in illness is as yet answered. Further measurement is necessary to address this question.

Nursing is a part of the social phenomenon of caring, which includes *compadrazgo,* with its unique features. While the practice of *compadrazgo* has been almost wholly embedded in informal social networks, with a partial tie to social-institutional religious practices, modern nursing has taken place almost exclusively within bureaucratized institutional and community agencies. This has limited the humanistic portions of the caring activities nurses have rendered to the extent that nurses are perceived in different ways by the public, but also by other health workers and nursing groups. Such a situation acts as a chronic deterrent to the impact that nursing could have on social welfare and may well threaten nursing's future viability, for it is often difficult to determine, even empirically, whether nursing caring activities make a difference in the well-being of people.

According to Leininger's comprehensive list of "Major Taxonomic Caring Constructs," which currently number 27, there are only four that can be considered with some assurance to be generally practiced by nurses, ie, Health Consultative Acts, Health Instruction Acts, Health Maintenance Acts, and Surveillance.[17] These are instrumental functions implicit in aspects of nursing curricula and in institutional and agency job descriptions. The remaining caring constructs identified by Leininger, for example, Compassion, Tenderness, Stress Alleviation, and 23 others, may be likewise implicitly included in nursing education and practice, but they are often left to the whims and personal inclinations of the individual nurse. The vague expectations and applications of care constructs lead to ambiguous behavior and norms. They tend to erode care as an explicit and important part of nursing. Mental health counselors, patient advocates, non-nurse physician assistants, patient educators, and community health counselors may use these care concepts as they deal with clients' weight, smoking, and stress concerns. The use of computerized surveillance for high-technology treatments in both institutional and outpatient settings will also detract from nurses' giving explicit care in a therapeutic and personalized way.

Professional nurses need to learn that both instrumental and affective components of caring compromise are the best way to help people. Flexibility is essential for endurance, as with *compadrazgo,* which has changed form in relation to differing socioenvironmental and cultural pressures. Interestingly, *compadrazgo* has not changed its essential function—to provide for an extension of close ties that yield the promise of both affective and instrumental sustenance to the cultural groups. While nursing may appear to be flexible owing to changes in this century, these changes have been limited. "Modern" nursing changes have largely been due to technologic innovations in highly complex treatment institutions, where the bulk of nurses have practiced. These changes have tended to support more instrumental care with limited humanitarian focus.

It is difficult to organize research activities that will prove relevant to nursing practice, for a wide gap continues to be perpetuated between an "ideal" image of nursing caring, which is eclectic in definition, and the actual practice of nursing, which is necessarily task-oriented. Nurses tend to respond to institutional pressures. Accordingly, *compadrazgo* should be subjected to more rigorous research in order to answer precise questions of its mediating effects in illness. Nursing care activities should also be subjected to greater precision in measurement related to the concept of *compadrazgo.* This may be difficult to study until some consensus is reached regarding an institutional compatibility between ideal and cognitive nursing care activities and functions.

REFERENCES

1. Leininger M (ed): Caring: An Essential Human Need. Proceedings of Three National Caring Conferences. Thorofare, NJ, Charles B. Slack, Inc., 1981.
2. Leininger M: Care: The Essence of Nursing. Thorofare, NJ, Charles B. Slack, Inc., 1983.
3. Leininger M: Caring: the essence and central focus of nursing. American Nurses' Foundation (Nursing Research Reports) 12(1):2, 13, 1977.
4. Fox R: Kinship and Marriage. Middlesex, England, Penguin Books, 1967.
5. Graburn N (ed): Readings in Kinship and Social Structure. New York, Harper and Row, 1971.
6. Levi-Strauss C: The Elementary Structures of Kinship. Bell JH, Von Sturmer IR, Needham R (trans). Boston, Beacon, 1969.
7. Mintz SW, Wolf ER: An analysis of ritual co-parenthood (compadrazgo). Southwest J Anthropol 6:341–368, 1950.
8. Davila M: Compadrazgo: fictive kinship in Latin America. *In* Graburn N (ed): Readings in Kinship and Social Structure. New York, Harper and Row, 1971, pp 396–406.
9. Dugan AB: Kin, Social Supports, and Depression Among Women of Mexican Heritage who are Single Parents. Ann Arbor, MI, University Microfilms, Int., 1983.
10. Leininger M: The phenomenon of caring: importance, research questions and theoretical considerations. *In* Leininger M (ed): Caring: An Essential Human Need. Proceedings of Three National Caring Conferences. Thorofare, NJ, Charles B. Slack, Inc., 1981, pp 3–15.
11. Sayers WC: Ritual kinship and negative effect. Am Sociol Rev 21:348–352, 1956.
12. Pearlin L, Schooler C: The structure of coping. J Health Soc Behavior 19(1):2–21, 1978.

13. Cobb S: Social support as a moderator of life stress. Psychosom Med 38:300–314, 1976.
14. Lin N, Simeone RS, Ensel WM, et al: Social support, stressful life events and illness: a model and an empirical test. J Health Soc Behavior 20(2):108–119, 1979.
15. Wallace AFC: Basic studies, applied projects, and eventual implementation: a case history of biological and cultural research in mental health. *In* Spindler GD (ed): The Making of Psychological Anthropology. Berkeley, CA, University of California Press, 1978, pp 203–216.
16. Spielberger CD, Gorsuch RL, Lushene RE: Manual for the State-Trait Anxiety Inventory (Self-Evaluation Questionnaire). Palo Alto, CA, Consulting Psychologists Press, 1970.
17. Nie NH, Hull CH, Jenkins JG, et al: SPSS: Statistical Package for the Social Sciences. 2nd ed. New York, McGraw-Hill, 1975.
18. Leininger M: Some philosophical, historical and taxonomic aspects of nursing and caring in American culture. *In* Leininger M (ed): Caring: An Essential Human Need. Proceedings of Three National Caring Conferences. Thorofare, NJ, Charles B. Slack, Inc., 1981, pp 133–143.

14

Caretaker-Child Interaction Observed in Two Appalachian Clinics

INTRODUCTION

Contact stimulation and caretaking behaviors are well-known variables important to the developmental status of infants and young children. Social scientists and others continue to be interested in the contribution of the culture to the personality development of children. Perhaps no other factor is as influential as the childrearing practices used by parents in shaping and patterning the children's cultural, psychosocial, and emotional development.

Spitz, using the tests and procedures worked out by Hertzer and Wolf, studied 130 children, 61 in a foundling home and 69 in a nursery.[1,2] The significant differences between the two institutions were as follows: The foundling home had few toys; and the children were isolated and virtually screened from the world, lying supine in the hollow of their mattress and lacking all human contact for most of the day, particularly from the age of three months onward. The nursery, on the other hand, provided each child with a mother surrogate who gave the child everything a good mother would. Spitz found that the developmental quotient of children in the foundling home occurred at approximately the same time that they were weaned. At this time, even the human contact they had during nursing terminated. Spitz concluded that it was the deprivation of maternal care, maternal stimulation, and maternal love that produced the clear evidence of damage to the foundling home infants, and that even when put in a more favorable environment at age 15 months, the psychosomatic damage could not be repaired by normal measures.[3]

The presence of "critical developmental periods" or "sensitive conditions" in early life has been demonstrated in many species, particularly in relation to the imprinting of birds and mammals.[4-6] These phenomena have also been identified

195

in primates. Harlow, for example, found early contact, through clinging, to be a primary factor that binds the mother and infant monkey.[7] The earliest tactile stimulation seemed to play an important role in facilitating the attachment responses. Stimulus deprivation was found to have long-lasting effects, producing abnormal behaviors in monkey offspring. Bowlby suggested that lack of contact stimulation delays formation of early bonding and, later, the ability to form close attachments.[8] He described the following childhood problems as characteristic of children suffering from lack of early contact stimulation: "superficial relationships, no capacity to care for people, inaccessibility, no emotional response to a situation where it is normal . . . ."[8]

The amount of stimulation provided by the adults is one of the major determinants of the infant's behavior. For example, Provence and Lipton noted that the response of the parent contributes to the process differentiation in the infant's mental function.[9] The parent's repetition, labeling, and response to the baby's reactions to his environment, his feelings, and his vocalizations are important to his recogniton of himself, of other persons, and of his world. The mother appears to influence the development of speech through a process of "mutual imitation." Moreover, the mother's speech is "both a carrier of the emotions and an organizing influence on the infant's mental apparatus." The mother, through her way of responding to the infant in actions and, especially, in speech, identifies or "labels" for him many things such as people, toys, himself, his feelings and actions, and those of others. He comes to be able to identify many aspects of inner and outer realities because she provides the appropriate experiences.[10]

Contactual interactions during the postpartum period could enhance human caretaking behaviors, as suggested by Bradley.[11] He suggests that mothers who breast-feed their neonates immediately after birth, more readily recognize and differentiate their own infant's cries, and generally show more "attentiveness" to their infants than do mothers who have delayed putting infants to the breast or have bottle-fed them. Klaus, Jerauld, and Kreger conducted a study of the importance of early contact between mother and full-term infants in the development of human maternal behaviors.[12] They found significant effects of "extended contact" in an experimental group of bottle-feeding mothers who were given an hour of interaction with their infants at three hours postpartum, plus 15 additional hours in the next three or four days. In contrast to the control group, the "extended contact" group evidenced greater soothing behaviors, more responsiveness to the infant's cries, and more attentiveness during the first-month examination.

The infant does not simply develop in response to the environment. Moss contends that maternal behavior seems initially to be under the control of the stimulus and reinforcing conditions provided by the young infant in such a way that at first the mother is shaped by the infant, which later facilitates her shaping the behavior of the child.[13] Roberson found that eye-to-eye contact seems to foster positive maternal feelings.[14] The mothers feel "being recognized" by the infant in a highly personal and intimate way is important. Perhaps this is a reason why mothers of blind children often feel rebuffed at first, for these mothers have been found to feel rejected by their infants.[15] Bowlby believes that the smiling of an infant acts as a social release of instinctual responses in the mother, along with such other innate "releasers" as crying, following, clinging, and sucking.[8] Lorenz goes so far as to suggest that the human smile is also a ritualized form of aggression, comparable with the "greeting" ceremonies that inhibit intraspecific fighting in many lower animals.[16]

The abovementioned studies have relevance to the caring theories formulated by Leininger.[17] According to Leininger: "Caring has long been expressed by human cultures throughout the history of humankind. Care, I believe, was essential for human growth, development, and survival," and "caring appears to be an extremely important and generic construct in human services."[17] Leininger considers caring as the central unifying concept and essence of nursing theory and practice. She states that caring makes nursing unique and different in form, expression, and content from other health care disciplines. She further suggests that caring is the primary focus of nursing, in contrast to medicine's unique and primary focus on curing processes, behaviors, and practices. She challenges nurses to identify, define, classify, and refine ethnocaring constructs, with the goal of gaining and using cultural and subcultural values, health habits, caring practices, and other culture-specific characteristics.

The following caring concepts from Leininger's ethnonursing and nursing constructs were expanded and further developed in order to quantify the behavioral interaction between the caretaker and the child. Leininger's caring constructs—such as comfort, concern, coping behaviors, facilitating, involvement, love, nurture, presence, protective behaviors, stimulation behaviors, stress alleviation, support, tenderness, touching, and trust—were categorized into five broad areas and operationally defined in order to quantify the observed caretaker-child interactional behaviors. The five categories are: proximity (distance), caretaking, pacifying, retrieval, and punishing behaviors.

METHOD

Overview

Mothers and fathers were randomly observed interacting with their children at two outpatient health clinics in an Appalachian county located in West Virginia. The author and another researcher independently observed behaviors of 122 caretaker-child pairs for a range of 16 to 30 minutes. A time-sampling procedure of one minute of observation followed by one minute of recording was used. Average reliability based on 12 checks was 81% with a range of 76% to 84%. Categories of caretaker-child behaviors observed by the researchers included proximity, caretaking, pacifying, retrieval, and punishing behaviors (Table 14-1).

Table 14-1. Categories of Caretaker-Child Behaviors

Categories	Caretaker-Child Behaviors
I. Proximity	Distance of children and their caretakers within 6 feet, out of 6 feet, and/or out of sight.
II. Caretaking	Offering food, clothing (putting on or removing), bodily needs, touching, soothing, holding hands or arm.
III. Pacifying	Caretaker presents child with toys, plays with the child, verbalizes with the child, child interacts with other child, caretaker holds child in arm or on lap.
IV. Retrieval	Verbal retrieval, physical retrieval.
V. Punishment	Loud verbalization, grabbing, slapping, shaking and roughly sitting the child.

Subjects

The samples of this study were randomly selected in two health clinics. The following criterion was applied: All caretaker-child pairs were composed of one or more children and a major caretaker waiting to be seen by the doctors in the two clinics designated as observational sites. The employees at both clinics indicated that the client population in Clinic A included approximately 60% of families not on public assistance, 20% of families who rely on public assistance, and approximately 20% of non-Appalachian families (those who were not born and raised in Appalachian regions, which included foreign-born immigrants). Clinic B was primarily serving the low-income Appalachian families. Although the purpose of this study was to concentrate on the Appalachian population, the design of the study prevented the researchers from assuring that the subjects observed were Appalachian. However, according to the informants, the majority (as high as 80%) of the middle- and low-income families still came to Clinic A for their health needs, and 95% of low-income Appalachians utilized Clinic B. For this study, except for those clients whose physical features, language, and other obvious cultural traits indicated that they were of other ethnic groups, those caretaker-child pairs with no identifiable information to indicate membership in other cultural groups were operationally defined as Appalachians.

The ages of the children observed in this study were estimated to be one month to six years old. Ninety-two mothers and 30 fathers were observed as primary caretakers of their children. The mothers' ages were estimated to be 16 to 40 years old. None of the teenage mothers' male partners were present at the two clinics.

Of the 30 fathers observed, most were estimated as 25 to 45 years old. Many caretakers had other adults or children who accompanied them to the clinics. Most frequently observed accompanying caretakers were the caretakers' spouses and siblings of the children.

Description of Time-Sampling Observations

The author and another researcher had a clipboard and stopwatch, and recorded the occurence of behaviors within a 30-minute period. In each minute, ratings would be made if behavior occurred either in the first 10 seconds or in the last 10 seconds. Each behavior defined in the observational checklist could be rated only once in a 60-second interval. The time-sampling procedure was one minute of observation followed by one minute of recording, for a maximum of 30 minutes per caretaker-child pair.

Procedure

The observers situated themselves in a corner of the designated clinics' waiting areas, where children and their caretakers came regularly for checkups, minor outpatient consultation, or treatment of various childhood diseases. All physical stimulation that occurred was recorded by the observers on the tool used for this study. All observed caretakers and their children were sitting in the waiting areas, and the observers placed themselves within 6 to 12 feet of the caretaker-child pairs in the settings. A time-sampling of one minute followed by one minute of recording was used. The researchers did not communicate verbally or nonverbally with the caretakers or children in the setting. The researchers pretended that they were parents waiting to see the doctor and doing their own reading or writing, without verbally communicating with the caretakers or the children. If the children approached the researchers and attempted to communicate with them, they were ignored by the researchers and soon were retrieved by their caretakers.

The subjects observed in this study were identified as a number on the checklist. Since the qualitative data were on a separate sheet with only the number from the checklist as identification, no portion of the data on the checklist or qualitative data on the separate sheet was identifiable to the individual subject observed.

Collection of Qualitative Data

Following observation of each caretaker-child pair, the interactional patterns were qualitatively recorded as accurately as possible in the form of an observational protocol on another sheet. The data were collected prospectively and retrospectively; the entire data were reviewed; and major behavioral themes were identified.

Observer Reliability

All observations were made by trained observers. The author and another observer independently noted a wide range of the parents' and children's behaviors by using a prepared checklist. These behavioral categories are listed in Table 14-1. The tool used to study the behaviors of caretaker-child pairs was first developed by Wurst and was modified by the author.[18] The tool was tested for reliability and face validity by using the judgment of independent observers. Observer reliability was computed by arranging for several observational sessions at the clinic. On these occasions, two observers independently dictated accounts of the caretaker-child pairs' behaviors. Correlational coefficients were computed to indicate the total number of occurrences of each behavior reported by one observer that were correctly reported by the other. Average reliability based on 12 checks was 81%, with a range of 76% to 84%. Approximately 30% of the transcripts of qualitative data was independently recorded by a coder other than the author, and the coder did not know that reliability was being assessed. Approximately 96% of reliability was obtained when two coders compared their results (Table 14-1).

The observers were able to observe approximately four to six caretaker-child pairs in a four-hour period. Because Clinic A was utilized by approximately one-fourth of the low-income Appalachian clients, and because they always came to Clinic A on a certain weekday except for emergencies, it was fairly easy for the clerk to identify subjects who were relying on public assistance. At the end of the observational period, the clerks went through all the recorded data and independently identified the low-income subjects by placing an X on the checklist and qualitative data sheets. The qualitative data, together with the observational checklist, were given to two trained coders, who transcribed all the behavioral items into numbers for computer analysis. Thus, the observers did not know which subjects were relying on public assistance and avoided possible observer bias. This precaution was not necessary when the data were collected in Clinic B, because the majority of clients were from low-income families.

Analysis of the Data

Data concerning the caretaker-child interaction were analyzed by using canned computer programs from SPSS (Statistical Package for the Social Sciences). A series of "t" tests and analysis of variance procedures were used to compare two or more groups to see whether the differences between group means were large enough to assume that the corresponding population means were different. Along with the quantitative analysis, cultural data derived from the observation, interviews of the health professionals in the clinics, and literature reviews were added to the interpretation of the data in this study.

RESULTS

Table 14-2 shows that there was a significant difference in the caretaker-child pairs between paying and public assistance groups. The caretakers in the group not receiving public assistance had fewer interactions within six feet of their children, and the public assistance caretakers exhibited more interactions with their children at distances greater than six feet. When comparing mother and father as primary caretakers, there were no statistical differences in terms of the caretakers' proximity to their children (Tables 14-2 and 14-3).

Analysis of variance was used to compare interactions in mother-daughter, mother-son, father-daughter, and father-son dyads. The data indicated that there were no statistical differences among the top four groups in terms of caretakers and their children's proximity from each other (Table 14-4).

Caretaking

When comparing caretakers from paying and public assistance groups in terms of caretaking behaviors, the data show that there were no significant differences between these two groups (Table 14-3). However, mothers tended to provide more contacts categorized as "caretaking behaviors" to their children. Mothers also provided a similar frequency of contact stimulation to daughters and sons, while fathers generally provided fewer contacts both to daughters and sons. Because there were only eight father-daughter dyads, Sheffel's multiple range test shows that no two groups are significantly different at the 0.05 level.

Pacifying

When comparing caretakers from paying and public assistance groups, there were no significant differences found between the two in terms of providing pacifying contacts to their children (Table 14-3). However, there was a significant difference when comparing mother with father as a primary caretaker of the child. The mothers tended to provide more pacifying contact stimulations to their charges than the fathers ($t=2.97$, $df=118$, $p<0.004$).

Analysis of variance shows that mothers tended to provide significantly more pacifying contacts with daughters than with sons. The fathers, on the other hand, provided fewer contacts to their children when compared with the mothers' behaviors. There were no differences in the fathers' contacts between daughter and son; they gave similar attention in this category (Table 14-7).

Punishing

In general, there were fewer contact responses in this category provided by the caretakers. Table 14-2 shows that in comparison with other behavioral contacts in the summary table, punishing contacts occurred less frequently among the

Text continues on p. 205.

Table 14-2. Summary Table of Mean and Standard Deviation of Caretaker-Child's Behaviors Recorded Per Minute of Observation for 122 Pairs

Behavior Contacts	Mean	Standard Deviation	Minimum	Maximum	Variance
Proximity					
Within 6 ft.	10.18	3.96	0.00	15.00	15.63
> 6 ft.	1.42	2.65	0.00	14.00	7.00
Out of sight	0.05	0.25	0.00	2.00	0.06
Caretaking					
Offering food to child	1.68	2.95	0.00	13.00	8.68
Clothing	0.79	1.26	0.00	6.00	1.57
Bodily needs	1.11	2.01	0.00	9.00	4.03
Touching	3.81	4.13	0.00	25.00	17.01
Soothing	3.64	4.80	0.00	15.00	22.96
Hold hands or arms	1.12	3.12	0.00	14.00	9.71
Pacifying					
Offer toys/play with toys	1.67	3.25	0.00	14.00	10.59
Play with child	1.86	3.43	0.00	15.00	11.79
Verbalize with child	5.25	5.00	0.00	15.00	25.25
Read to child	0.42	1.40	0.00	8.00	1.98
Child play/interact	2.40	3.97	0.00	15.00	15.75
On lap or arm	4.68	5.50	0.00	15.00	30.24
Punishing					
Loud verbalization	0.29	1.09	0.00	6.00	1.18
Grabbing child	0.14	0.66	0.00	4.00	0.44
Slapping child	0.06	0.37	0.00	3.00	0.05
Shaking child	0.03	0.22	0.00	2.00	0.05
Roughly sitting	0.08	0.42	0.00	3.00	0.18
Physical retrieval	0.15	0.59	0.00	3.00	0.34
Child's Other Behavior					
Child cry/unhappy	0.70	1.53	0.00	7.00	2.33
Child asleep	0.34	1.44	0.00	9.00	2.08
Adult's Other Behavior					
Concentrate on reading	0.53	1.83	0.00	9.00	3.34
Talking to adult	4.71	4.32	0.00	15.00	18.66
Gentle verbal retrieval	0.22	0.94	0.00	6.00	0.86

Source: Prepared by Janet Wang

Table 14-3. Comparison of Caretaker-Child Behaviors in Non-Public Assistance and Public Assistance Groups

Variable Behavioral Contact Observed	Number of Cases	Mean	Standard Deviation	F Value	2-Tailed Prob.	Polled Variance Estimate		
						T Value	DF	2-Tailed Prob.
Proximity Within 6 ft.								
Non-Public Assistance	81	11.1481	3.366	1.36	0.281	-2.25	120	0.026*
Public Assistance	41	12.5366	2.882					
> 6 ft.								
Non-Public Assistance	81	0.0123	0.111	12.94	0.000	-2.31	120	0.023*
Public Assistance	41	0.1220	0.400					
Caretaking								
Non-Public Assistance	81	12.9506	14.495	1.98	0.019	0.94	120	0.348
Public Assistance	41	10.5610	10.301					
Pacifying								
Non-Public Assistance	81	16.4321	15.201	1.30	0.359	0.13	120	0.898
Public Assistance	41	16.0732	13.316					
Punishing								
Non-Public Assistance	81	0.1235	0.509	73.00	0.000	-3.94	120	0.000**
Public Assistance	41	2.0488	4.353					

*p < 0.05
**p < 0.01
Source: Prepared by Janet Wang

Table 14-4. Comparison of Caretaker-Child's Behaviors in Father or Mother as a Primary Caretaker

Variable Behavioral Contact Observed	Number of Cases	Mean	Standard Deviation	F Value	2-Tailed Prob.	Polled Variance Estimate		
						T Value	DF	2-Tailed Prob.
Proximity								
Within 6 ft.								
Mother	90	11.6778	3.215	1.14	0.618	0.69	118	0.490
Father	40	11.2000	3.438					
> 6 ft.								
Mother	90	0.0667	0.292	0.0000	1.0000	1.25	118	0.215
Father	30	0.0000	0.0000	0.0000				
Caretaking								
Mother	90	14.033	13.571	1.69	0.109	2.97	118	0.004**
Father	30	5.9667	10.430					
Pacifying								
Mother	90	18.411	14.997	1.77	0.082	2.97	118	0.004**
Father	30	9.5333	11.258					
Punishing								
Mother	90	0.9444	2.981	3.29	0.001	1.13	118	0.262
Father	30	0.3000	1.643					

*p < 0.05
**p < 0.01
Source: Prepared by Janet Wang

Table 14-5. Analysis of Variance Summary Table for Caretaker-Child's Behaviors in Mother-Daughter, Mother-Son, Father-Daughter, and Father-Son Pairs

Source of Variation	DF	Sum of Square	Mean Square	F-Ratio	F-Prob.
Proximity					
Within 6 ft.					
Between Groups	3	18.5707	6.1902	0.575	0.6326
Within Groups	116	1249.0210	10.7674		
> 6 ft.					
Between Groups	3	0.1008	0.0336	0.513	0.6742
Within Groups	116	7.5992	0.0655		
Caretaking					
Between Groups	3	1527.8223	509.2741	3.032	0.0321*
Within Groups	116	19482.1444	167.9495		
Pacifying					
Between Groups	3	2130.4551	710.1517	3.530	0.0171*
Within Groups	116	23334.1363	201.1563		
Punishing					
Between Groups	3	10.5804	3.5268	0.471	0.7208
Within Groups	116	867.7863	7.4809		

*$p < 0.05$
Source: Prepared by Janet F. Wang

caretaker-child dyads observed in this study. A series of "t" tests indicated that caretakers who rely on public assistance tended to punish more frequently than their paying counterparts. However, when comparing mother with father as a primary caretaker, there were no significant differences between the two parents. Table 14-5 further indicates that there are no differences in this behavior when comparing father-son, father-daughter, mother-son, and mother-daughter interaction.

DISCUSSION

That the measurement of caretaker-child interactions can be made and studied in different settings or clinics was demonstrated in this report. Since there was no verbal or nonverbal communication required to collect the behavioral data about the interactions, the researchers can use the behavioral checklist to document behavior of the caretaker-child pairs in different settings.

The study found significant differences in the proximity of contact stimulations provided by public assistance and paying caretaker groups. Although this was an observational study in which there were no data that provided causal links, the assumption was that this study served as a snapshot to describe and capture the essence of the caretaker-child interactions in this Appalachian subculture.

One of the limitations of this study was that the researcher did not know the socioeconomic status of the client population, and analysis of the data was severely limited by separating the two populations into those who rely on public assistance and those who don't. Those who do not rely on public assistance were operationally defined as middle class. Another limitation was the setting for the observation. Although there were several caretaker-child pairs who came into the clinic, these middle-class caretakers would not wait for the doctors. The waiting area of Clinic A was especially small in that only about 10 to 12 people could be comfortably accommodated. Many clients complained that it gave them claustrophobia. The small space and long waiting period offered an especially rich opportunity for the researcher to observe the parent-child interactions. The small space was also an advantage for the researcher because she could see the interaction easily. The limitation was that not all parents waited there, and therefore many opportunities to observe may have been missed.

The middle-class caretakers tended to be impatient, often looking at their watches and pacing the floor while waiting for the doctor. However, it was this group of caretakers who often brought with them educational toys, books, and nutritious food. They tended to supervise their children's activities closely. They managed to occupy their children with various activities in those short periods of waiting, usually no more than 30 to 40 minutes. Mothers often read to their children, worked with them on writing and spelling, or explained things in detail. They also brought crackers, cereal in a bowl, juices in thermoses, or raisins and fruits as snacks for their children.

On the other hand, the low-income mothers seldom brought toys, books, or nutritious food with them. They were less likely to read to the children or entertain them with toys. They tended to be more preoccupied. Some mothers whose own teeth were missing would bring candies, coke, chewing gum, and cookies to eat. The author believed that the mother's missing teeth were a result of a lack of knowledge and possibly the inability to afford the cost of dental services.

The middle-class caretakers were more rigid and firm in terms of what the children were allowed to have for snacks. When one clerk at the clinic offered a lollipop, the children of the middle-class group appeared to be surprised and expressed great excitement, but they were disappointed when their mothers forbade them to have the treat. On one occasion, the researcher noted that after the clerk offered a lollipop to a young child, his mother angrily snapped at the clerk, "Don't ever do that again! We don't have junk food like that. He doesn't know what that is."

When a lollipop was offered to a low-income child, he went right to the clerk to get more and demanded to have other flavors. The mothers of these children did not stop their children's consumption of candy, as the middle-class mothers did. They appeared to be more relaxed and permissive in regard to eating candy in the clinic.

Some who have studied the Appalachian poor would say that even if the mother did not want her child to have the candy, she would not feel that she had the right to disagree with the authority figures.

Weller has written much about what he terms a parental attitude of permissiveness and indulgence that is held by mountain parents toward their children. Weller found:

> Children are seldom required to do what they do not want to do. I have known of sick children who, on finding their medicine distasteful, were allowed not to take it, even though their welfare depended upon their doing so. If a child wants candy or pop he can have it, even though his teeth may be rotting out because of it. If a child does not particularly want to have a new experience (going to camp, for example), parents seldom urge him to go for the good it might do him. They let the child make the decision.[19]

Researchers have found that malnutrition reduces the child's responsiveness to stimulation, and this reduced responsiveness itself can induce apathy in the adult who is caring for the child. The child appears to add to his own disadvantaged environment.[20] Many mothers in the lower socioeconomic group are often young and inexperienced, and they offer a different kind of mothering to an infant.[10] Marked class differences have been found in child-rearing practices, although the research findings are conflicting. For example, Sears, Maccoby, and Lewin found that middle-class mothers are more permissive than those of the lower class, while Havinghurst concluded that middle-class mothers are more restrictive.[21,22] Whiting and Child found that children of the American middle class are among the most restricted of anywhere in the world.[23]

This researcher also noted that children from the middle class tend to be more self-assured and confident. They would ask questions and have verbal arguments with siblings. The children would fight and bang on the door. If the clerk came to ask them to stop, they would involve the clerk in the play-fight situations. When the clerk threatened, "I am going to call your mother," the children replied, "I don't care." These children were not able to adjust to the tight space of the small waiting area and were very active in the room.

On the other hand, the low-income children were especially polite and respectful of authority. Their mothers were very polite to the clerk and the staff, as if the staff had given them favors. Very often the mothers expressed appreciation of the care given by the clinic. One clerk remarked, "Middle-class mothers behave like you owe them something, and when the appointments run slow, they upset easily. The low-income mothers would sit patiently and wait for their turn." The low-income children, in general, were well-behaved, as evidenced by the quantitative data in which low-income children were punished more frequently than the middle-class children. The mothers of low-income children often reminded their children to sit quietly: "Sit here, I will be right back," and the children would sit quietly without problems. These children seemed to obey their parents and have respect for their authority.

In socially and culturally deprived homes, there is usually little space and few toys or books. One school teacher revealed that some of the low-income children did not know what a book was, never having been exposed to books or other objects normally found in a middle-class home. Low-income parents perhaps are preoccupied with their problems and may have little energy to invest in their children's achievements.

Perhaps no other area reflected the differences between the two groups as greatly as verbal skills. The middle-class children tend to have more verbal interaction with adults. They would greet the nurse and staff and engage them in conversation. They seemed to be more in control of themselves and wanted to be informed about what was expected of them in the clinic visit. When their younger siblings went into the examining room, the children quickly asked the adult what the nurse or doctor would do to their sister or brother. They tended to identify with their siblings closely and wanted to be informed. The caretakers of these children would go to great extents to explain what seemed to be a complicated medical process to the young child. The mother would use positive terms to explain to the child. One five-year-old demanded that the nurse explain what she was going to do with his sister. "You are not going to hurt her, are you?", he asked.

The middle-class mothers appeared to be more interested in communicating with their children either verbally or nonverbally. Mothers of infants often played nonverbal facial games in which they mimicked smiling or crying faces. There was a continuous display of different facial expressions. It appeared that the mother was the best entertainment for the infant, and she interacted with her child quietly and intensely. Low-income mothers, especially the teenage mothers, showed far fewer intense facial interactions with their infants. One teenage mother accompanied by her own mother exhibited low bonding behaviors with her infant. She interacted with her infant minimally, while the maternal grandmother took over the caretaking chores.

Perhaps the socialization procedures typically employed in the middle-class families were likely to encourage the child to perceive reality in terms of more than one alternative. The caretakers provided a range of positive interpretations to the child. Furthermore, these interactions may also create anxiety and uncertainty as the child learns to interpret by himself. Not only is he made aware of a range of possible interpretations, but he is also expected to make an individual interpretation of the situations to which he is exposed.

Berinstein and Henderson found that: (1) the middle-class mothers are more likely than working-class mothers to respond to the child's attempt to interact verbally with the mother in a range of contexts; (2) the middle-class mothers are less likely to use coercive methods of control; and (3) the middle-class mothers are more likely to explain to the child why they want a change in behavior.[24] It appears that the middle-class children acquire language skills in such a way that the child has access to both operation and principles. They tend to regulate their own learning in an arranged environment which encourages autonomy in learning.

Another interesting observation was the quick interchange between mothers at Clinic A, where most of the clients are of middle-class background. The mothers were interested in other children and often complimented them. Verbal exchanges were mainly information-giving, mimicking, and support of each other. They exchanged eye contact and comments on each other's caretaking experiences, and quickly went into self-disclosure of some very personal information. Perhaps women, in general, are warmer, more empathic, and more interested in other women's caretaking experiences and related problems. Rapport seemed to be established quickly and proceeded to self-disclosure of personal feelings. Female caretakers observed in Clinic A tended to display support, self-disclosure, and pleasantness to each other.

Observation at Clinic B, where most of the low-income caretakers were, showed a different picture. Caretakers sat quietly and mainly kept to themselves. They whispered to their children or talked to their husbands, wives, or mothers in low voices. The self-disclosure and quick verbal interchange with strangers observed in Clinic A were not seen at Clinic B. Perhaps the client population was different, and the low-income caretakers were not feeling confident and comfortable enough to self-disclose to strangers.

On many occasions, the researcher observed that some low-income mothers appeared unkempt and wore soiled clothes into Clinic A. Perhaps because of the small waiting area, it seemed especially difficult for the other people to tolerate noticeable odor. At times, the staff would take the mother into the examining room and remove her from the rest of the clients. One mother in particular brought several of her ten children to the clinic. It was a chilling winter day, and the children were poorly dressed with torn clothes; a few of them had no shoes. Young children were left for the older children to care for, and the mother was not sensitive to her young children's needs. The crying and fussing of the young children did not appear to bother the mother. This researcher gave credit to this mother, however, for as poor as she was, she was able to come to the clinic for her health needs. Perhaps she had no babysitter, a situation that would make it necessary for her to bring the entire family to the clinic. She may have gone through many difficult arrangements in order to get transportation for the whole family to the clinic. Perhaps there was also no running water in the home; in these circumstances, water would be too precious for her to clean the children and herself. The author strongly believes that the Appalachian poor have many constraints. Physical, socioeconomic, cultural, and educational factors in our society clearly have a significant impact upon the development of the child, and no study of the development of an individual is complete without an understanding of these factors.

Male caretakers tended to verbalize less and engaged in less eye contact with other clients in the waiting area. They would engage in reading, staring at the ceiling, or looking at their shoes or the floor, seeming to concentrate on their own thinking. It appeared that the male caretakers were uncomfortable in such a setting, where the majority of the clients were mothers. They appeared to be left out and engaged in minimal verbal exchange with other clients in the waiting area. Even when several of the mothers were engaging in discussion, the male caretakers remained quiet without joining the group discussion.

They also did not participate in interaction with their children. Often they would bury their heads in books and magazines, and when the children asked questions, they answered selectively. This qualitative assessment was supported by the quantitative analysis, in that significant differences between mothers' and fathers' behaviors were noted (Table 14-6). One father, also a physician, never came into the waiting area; instead, he paced back and forth in the hallway, holding his son in his arms, and verbalized minimally. One father was so uncomfortable with children that he failed to sense the high temperature in the room, and the child wore a coat until the mother came in and removed it. The mothers tended to display greater nonverbal communication with their children. The mothers tended to repeat, label the objects, and respond to their children with more words than the fathers. Many mothers mimicked words with their babies and allowed the baby to explore their faces. The mothers actively responded to their children and used a greater number of adjectives to identify feelings.

It is also interesting to observe how creative the caretaker can be. One mother removed her jacket and put it on her three-year-old girl, starting to role-play with her. It was amazing to observe the richness of the child's vocabulary when the mother and daughter continued to exchange verbally. This type of verbal exchange was not observed among the father-child dyads. Although the subjects to be observed were randomly selected, there were three times more father-son than father-daughter dyads. Perhaps fathers have more concerns for and feel vulnerable about their sons' illnesses and want to be with them in person.

Analysis of variance was used to compare behaviors of mother- and father-child interactions. The data show that there are significant differences between mothers and fathers interacting with their children. The quantitative data also support the qualitative assessment in that fathers spent approximately six minutes caretaking their children, while mothers spent twice that time. The data also indicate that mothers spent more time caretaking their daughters than their

Table 14-6. Analysis of Variance for Caretaking Behaviors in Mother-Daughter, Mother-Son, Father-Daughter, and Father-Son Pairs

Source of Variation	DF	Sum of Square	Mean Square	F-Ratio	F-Prob.
		Summary of ANOVA			
Caretaking					
Between Groups	3	1527.82	509.27	3.032	0.0321*
Within Groups	116	19482.14	167.95		
Total	119	21009.97			

*p < 0.05

Mean and Standard Deviation

Source of Variance	N	Mean	Standard Deviation	Minimum	Maximum	95% Conf. Int. for Mean
Caretaking						
Mother-Daughter	43	14.90	13.34	0.00	57.00	10.80 to 19.01
Mother-Son	47	13.23	13.87	0.00	43.00	9.16 to 17.31
Father-Daughter	8	6.25	.72	0.00	17.00	−0.21 to 12.71
Father-Son	22	5.86	11.41	0.00	45.00	0.80 to 10.93
Total	120	12.02	13.29	0.00	57.00	9.61 to 14.42

Test for homogeneity of variances
   Cochran's C = Max. Variance/Sum (Variances) = 0.34, P = 0.23 (Approx.)
   Bartlett-Box F = 1.260, F = 0.29
   Maximum Variance/Minimum Variance = 3.23

Multiple Range Test use of Scheffe procedure: No two groups are significantly different at 0.05 level.

Source: Prepared by Janet Wang

sons (Table 14–6). Perhaps mothers were more protective of their daughters than of their sons. Mothers also spent an average of four more minutes pacifying their daughters than they did their sons. There was no difference in paternal attention to either sex child.

In the study of father-child attachments, Lamb found that there are significant differences in the types of play and physical contact that infants have with their mothers and fathers—differences that are consistent across time.[25] The researcher contends that infants are attached to both parents early in life, and that the mother-infant and father-infant relationships differ qualitatively. The fact that the mother- and father-infant relationships involve different types of interaction is important, for it suggests that mothers and fathers provide babies with different kinds of experiences and, hence, that they probably have different roles to play in the child's social personality development. As attachment figures and sources of security, however, the two parents play similar roles in their children's development.

It appeared that children are attached from the earliest age to both parents, and that the two relationships differ qualitatively. Fathers are not merely mother-substitutes; they also interact with their children in unique and different ways. This makes it possible for the child to learn and grow with the aid of the two parents. It seemed that fathers are more comfortable with their sons and may be playing an especially important role in facilitating the development of the sex-role-appropriate behaviors in their sons.

The data show that the child's gender plays a role in modifying mothers' and fathers' patterns of interaction with the child. As a wide range of other studies has shown, fathers and mothers—from the newborn period onward—treat boys and girls differently.[26,27] Fathers generally show more involvement with their sons, while mothers show the complementary pattern of more involvement with their daughters.[28]

Redican's long-term laboratory study of male infant sex-pair differences in contact showed that they were more pronounced than in adult female-infant pairs. Male adults had more extensive contact with male children.

> Mothers tended to play with female infants whereas adult males did so with male infants. In general mothers interact more positively with female infants and adult males more with male infants.[29]

Finally, there were no differences found in punishing behaviors provided by the caretakers. In terms of actual numbers of contacts per minute of observation, the caretakers observed in this study demonstrated fewer punishing contacts in comparison with other behavioral categories (Table 14-7). However, there was a significant difference in punishing behavior—low-income mothers appeared to punish more frequently than the other caretakers.

Implication

The Appalachian poor are facing a hard time ahead. Although dealing with the many constraints of the Appalachian poor seems to be beyond nursing intervention, nurses indeed can be helpful and effective in caring for them. It is essential for the nurses who want to be change agents to learn about their client's cultural differences and similarities. When dealing with clients from various

Table 14-7. Analysis of Variance for Pacifying Behaviors in Mother-Daughter, Mother-Son, Father-Daughter, and Father-Son Pairs

Summary of ANOVA

Source of Variation	DF	Sum of Square	Mean Square	F-Ratio	F-Prob.
Pacifying					
Between Groups	3	2130.46	710.15	3.53	0.01*
Within Group	116	23334.14	201.16		
Total	119	25464.59			

*p < 0.05

Mean and Standard Deviation

Source of Variance	N	Mean	Standard Deviation	Minimum	Maximum	95% Conf. or Mean
Pacifying						
Mother-Daughter	43	20.49	16.24	0.00	61.00	15.49 to 25.49
Mother-Son	47	16.51	13.66	0.00	62.00	12.50 to 20.52
Father-Daughter	8	9.13	12.60	0.00	25.00	−1.41 to 19.66
Father-Son	22	9.68	11.05	0.00	39.00	4.78 to 14.58
Total	120	16.20	14.63	0.00	62.00	13.54 to 18.84

Test for homogeneity of variances
Cochran's C = Max. variance/Sum (Variance) = 0.36, P = 0.129 (Approx.)
Bartlett-Box F = 1.38, P = 0.248

Multiple Range Test use of Scheffe Procedure indicates a significant difference at the 0.050 level.

Source: Prepared by Janet Wang

socioeconomic backgrounds, the ethical principles employed must include the recognition of cultural differences and values of the cultural group involved.

It is extremely important for the Appalachians to trust the health workers.

> Whether a patient stays in a hospital or leaves against medical advice depends more on his personal relations with hospital personnel than on any understanding he may have of his medical condition and the hospital's technical competence in treating him.[30]

The fear of authority and person-oriented, rather than task-oriented, cultural values were also described by Weller, who found that outsiders or authority figures were perceived by the Appalachians with fear, antagonism, and suspicion.[19] Loofe reported that Appalachians often became anxious when they had to use services of unfamiliar organizations, such as the hospital or government agency offices.[31]

Ethnocentrism among the nurses can prevent them from effectively caring for the clients and meeting the clients' needs. Nurses must be especially sensitive, gentle, empathic, and patient in dealing with the Appalachian subcultural groups. Cultural relativity requires that the subcultural groups be judged on the basis of their own standards. Their belief system and standard of cleanliness are different from that of middle-class Americans. Since most of the professional health workers are of middle-class background, the use of middle-class standards to judge the Appalachian poor clients is a cultural imposition of their own belief system on the clients.

Nurses can give positive feedback to mothers who interact with and nurture their children well. Nurses should purposely approach the male caretakers and give positive recognition of their involvement with the caretaking of their children. The data show that the male caretakers appeared to be uncomfortable and felt out of place in the clinic, as observed by the researchers. The nurse can be a change agent by arranging and providing an atmosphere more comfortable to male caretakers by involving them in discussion and planning for the care of their children.

Finally, nurses must also be aware of the vastness of the teaching needs of the Appalachian poor. They must be aware, also, of the impossibility of meeting these needs in a short-term interaction. Therefore, there is a real need for long-term interaction, based on initial acceptance of the clients' different value system. Until the trust relationship can be established between the nurse and the clients, effective teaching cannot occur.

REFERENCES

1. Spitz RA: Hospitalization: an inquiry into the genesis of psychiatric conditions in early childhood. Psychoanalytic Study Child 1:53–74, 1945.
2. Hertzer H, Wolf K: Baby tests. Zeitschrift fur Psychologic, 1928, p 107.
3. Spitz RA: Hospitalization: a follow-up report. Psychoanalytic Study Child 2:113–117, 1946.
4. Lorenz KZ: Der kumpan in der umvelt des vogels. J Ornithol 83:137–214, 1935.

5. Hess E: Imprinting in birds. Science 146:1128–1139, 1964.
6. Slucking W: Imprinting and Early Learning. Chicago, Aldine Publishing Co., 1945.
7. Harlow HF, Hanson EM: The maternal affectional system of rhesus monkeys. *In* Rheingold HL (ed): Maternal Behavior in Mammals. New York, Wiley & Sons, Inc., 1963, pp 254–281.
8. Bowlby J: The nature of a child's tie to his mother. Int J Psychoanal 39:350–373, 1958.
9. Provence S, Lipton R: Infants in Institutions. New York, International University Press, Inc., 1962.
10. Lewis M: Clinical Aspects of Child Development. Philadelphia, Lea and Febiger, 1973, pp 17–35.
11. Bradley RA: Personal communication, 1973.
12. Klaus MH, Jerauld R, Kreger NP, et al: Maternal attachment: importance of the first postpartum days. N Engl J Med 286:460–463, 1972.
13. Moss HA: Sex, age and state as determinants of mother-infant interaction. Merrill-Palmer Q Behav Devel 13(1):19–36, 1967.
14. Roberson KS: The role of eye-to-eye contact in maternal-infant behavior. J Child Psychol Psych 8(1):13–25, 1967.
15. Fraiberg S: Paralleled and divergent patterns in blind and sighted infants. Psychoanalytic Study Child 23:264–300, 1968.
16. Lorenz K: On Aggression. New York, Harcourt, Brace and World, 1966.
17. Leininger M: The phenomenon of caring: importance, research questions and theoretical considerations. *In* Leininger M (ed): Caring: An Essential Human Need. Proceedings of the Three National Caring Conferences. Thorofare, NJ, Charles B. Slack, Inc., 1981, pp 133–143.
18. Wurst K: Caretaker-child interactions in Greek and American culture. Paper presenterd at the annual meeting of the Northeastern Educational Research Association, Allenville, New York, October 1978.
19. Weller JE: Yesterday's People: Life in Contemporary Appalachia. Lexington, University of Kentucky Press, 1966 p 66.
20. Cravioto J, DeLicardi ER, Birch HG: Nutrition, growth and neuro-integrative development: an experimental and ecologic study. Pediatrics 38:318, 1966.
21. Sears R, Maccoby E, Lewin H: Patterns of Child Rearing. Evanston, Illinois, Row, Peterson, 1957, p 15.
22. Havinghurst H, Wolf K: Father of the Man. Boston, Houghton Mifflin Co., 1947.
23. Whiting J, Child I: Child Training and Personality. New Haven, CT, Yale University Press, 1953, pp 106–118.
24. Berinstein B, Henderson D: Social class differences in the relevance of language to socialization. *In* Berinstein B (ed): Class Codes and Control, 1973, pp 24–78.
25. Lamb ME: Social interaction in infancy and the development of personality. *In* Lamb ME (ed): Social and Personality Development. New York, Holt, Rinehart and Winston, 1979, pp 230–259.
26. Rebelsky F, Hanks C: Fathers' verbal interaction with infants in the first three months of life. Child Devel 42:63–68, 1971.
27. Rendina I, Dicerscheid JD: Father involvement with first born infants. Family Coordinator 25:373–379, 1976.
28. Parke RD, Sawin DB: The fathers' role in infancy: a re-evaluation. Family Coordinator 25:365–371, 1976.
29. Redican WK: Adult male-infant interactions in nonhuman primates. *In* Lamb ME (ed): The Role of the Father in Child Development. New York, Wiley and Sons, 1976, pp 345-385.
30. Pearsall M: Communicating with the educationally deprived. *In* Mielke D (ed): Teaching Mountain Children. Boone, NC, Appalachian Consortium Press, 1978, pp 59–66.
31. Loofe D: Appalachians' Children. Lexington, Kentucky, The University of Kentucky Press, 1971, pp 60-75.

15

The Child's View of Chemically Induced Alopecia

Easing the psychosocial impact of hair loss or alopecia among children is a pervasive clinical problem for pediatric oncology nurses. This exploratory study utilizes ethnographic methods to learn how children conceptualize alopecia and to determine the sociocultural context in which these children experience hair loss following chemotherapy. The purpose of this research was to answer the question: What cultural knowledge guides the behavior of children when they lose their hair after being treated with chemotherapy for cancer?

The way in which human beings experience disfigurement and changes in body image can assist in understanding care behaviors, processes, and intervention modalities. A crucial need in clinical nursing research is descriptive accounts of health and illness experiences, care, and caretaking from the point of view of human beings.

This chapter is organized under the following headings: (1) the conceptual orientation; (2) the ethnographic methods of data collection and analysis; and (3) the findings, including the researcher-informant experience, domains of meaning relevant to the child's experience during hair loss, and cultural themes representing a holistic view of the cultural system of knowledge that guides the behavior of children with alopecia due to chemotherapy.

THE CONCEPTUAL ORIENTATION

The organizing ideas for this study are grounded in the constructs of culture, illness, societal values, and care (Table 15-1). The conceptual orientation for culture is found in the work of Goodenough, Spradley, and others who view culture as a cognitive system.[1-3] Culture is knowledge used by human beings (in our case, children) to interpret experience and generate behavior.[2] In this research, the cognitive conceptualization of culture focuses on the rules and principles for children's behavior during the experience of hair loss. These rules

Table 15-1. Conceptual Orientation for the Study of the Child's View of Alopecia

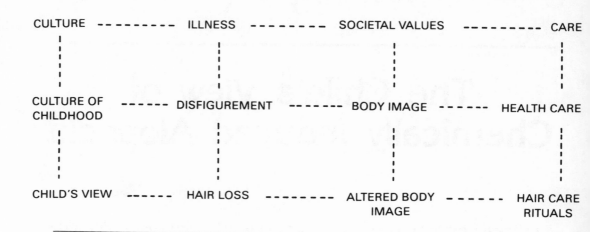

and principles are abstracted by the researcher from observational and interview data.

The culture of childhood has been conceptualized in the work of Goodman, Harre, Aamodt, and others.[4-7] The view of the child is recognized as different from the adult view. Furthermore, the child is perceived as a human being who views the social situation and selects and rejects, consciously and unconsciously, among alternatives available in the environment.

Illness, disfigurement, and hair loss are differing levels of abstraction referring to a nonnormal state of a human being—disfigurement being a characteristic of illness, and hair loss being a special case of disfigurement. The notion of societal values introduces the idea of how society serves as an audience to any and all human behavior—in this case, the concept of body image, or, more accurately, acceptable body image. An altered body image can be expected to accompany hair loss.[8]

The concept of care derives from the work of Leininger, Hyde, Aamodt, and Watson.[9-18] Care can be conceptualized as doing for self or doing for others.[17,19] For the purposes of this study, care is conceptualized as care of self. Thus, the study attempts to bring a different dimension to our understanding of the complexities in a child's self-care during an experience such as hair loss. Health care rituals represent kinds of caregiving activities of self and others, with hair care rituals as the object of the research.

METHODS

Participant observation and the ethnographic interview following the protocol of Spradley were the methods used for data collection and analysis.[2,3]

The study was conducted in a pediatric oncology clinic in a university hospital in the southwestern United States. Eight children, ages 7 to 17, who had or were experiencing hair loss were interviewed. Ethnographic interviews were used to discover domains of meaning and relationships among domains in the language of the children which reflected their definitions of reality. Each child was interviewed three to five times.

Beginning ethnographic questions, or grand tour questions were: What happened when you began to lose your hair? What did you do? What did others do?[2] Information collected during each interview was analyzed and used for generating questions for each succeeding interview. Domains of meaning were generated to develop a structure for the ethnographic data. Children were asked to validate the information during and after the analysis. Returning to the child following each interview and sharing with him how we had organized his linguistic labels and meanings helped assure the researchers that what had been collected was what the child wanted to say.

Ethnography field work is a reflexive activity; that is, the direction of the research is often guided by the knowledge, clues, and intuitive responses of the ethnographer. In this study, the researchers became participants during the process of interviewing as they established themselves with the child informant, and translated the child's language to a form meaningful for practice and research nurses. The researchers also became participants in the analysis when data from two or more children were combined. These activities are recognized methodologic problems in all ethnographic work.

THE FINDINGS

The findings are reported in a discussion of the researcher-informant experience, in ethnographic data reported in domains of meaning for the child with hair loss, and in cultural themes representing the researcher's view of the whole system of the culture of childhood during an experience of hair loss.

The Researcher-Informant Experience

Eight children and three interviewers participated in the data collection process. The children, four boys and four girls, were ages 7 to 17 years and had varying degrees of hair loss at the time of the interviews—from none to complete (Table 15-2). Two children were Mexican-American, and six were Anglo-American.

Children were selected because they were willing to talk about themselves. Whereas school-aged children up to the ages of 11 to 13 liked to talk to others about themselves, teenagers were often more reticent. However, one 15-year-old, who died soon after the interviews, wanted to help other children and for this reason felt a real need to tell what she knew. In her view, this was her unfinished business. Preschoolers were not as interested, not as committed, and more often shy.

Three graduate students who had participated in various ways in the nursing

Table 15-2. Informant Demographic Data

Diagnosis	Degree of Loss at Interview	Sex	Age	Ethnicity	Attending School	Head Covering
Acute Lymphocytic Leukemia (ALL)	None	M	12	Anglo	Yes	Baseball cap
Osteogenic Sarcoma	Complete	F	14	Anglo	No	Scarf or wig
Wilms' Tumor	Patches of sparse hair	M	7	Mex-Amer	No	Knitted cap
Ovarian Teratoma with Spinal Metastasis	Complete	F	11	Anglo	Yes	Scarf or wig
Osteogenic Sarcoma	80%	F	13	Anglo	Yes	Scarf or wig
CA Myelogenous Leukemia (CML)	None	M	17	Anglo	Yes	Cap or wig
Acute Lymphocytic Leukemia (ALL)	Small patches of hair loss on top of head	F	15	Mex-Amer	Yes	Baseball cap
Hodgkin's Disease	Complete	F	15	Mex-Amer	No	Scarf or wig

activities of the clinic conducted the ethnographic interviews. The first interview was devoted to getting to know the child, and most often direct questions were not asked until the second or third interview. In this study, researcher experiences that characterized the interviews were: (1) the frankness of the children; (2) the often intense emotional response of the interviewer to the circumstances of the children; (3) arranging the interviews within the busy clinic schedule; and (4) monitoring the child's tolerance for sensitive questions, energy use, and change in mood.

Many children recognized the purpose of telling their story. For example, one very ill teenager insisted on talking, although she was obviously fatigued, because she thought that this kind of information could help other children cope with the experience of hair loss. Frequently, children were very blunt in talking about names others called them and just how it felt to be bald. They recounted stories of what happened to them when they wore a wig, and they all had strong feelings about how they had not changed with the loss of their hair.

Interviewers were caring for other children in the clinics, and in these settings they were somewhat desensitized to what children with hair loss represented to them. When they first interviewed those selected for the study, however, they often felt awkward and hesitant about bothering children who were experiencing a pain-ridden body and pain-producing procedures. Interviews were conducted in the clinic, in the hospital, and at home. Home and hospital were more relaxed for both child and interviewer. Clinic interviews meant sandwiching 30 minutes here and there in between blood drawings, doctors' visits, test results, and chemotherapy. Nevertheless, when there was a choice between waiting or talking with the interviewer, children were ready to talk. How the child felt influenced the data collection process. For example, some children joked about the hair loss experience and what they would do about it if they could. A seven-year-old boy told how he picked hair that had fallen from his mother's head and pasted it on his own. Other children were delighted to be tape-recorded and to listen to their own voices.

Domains of Meaning in the Child's View of Hair Loss

Nine domains of meaning emerged from the data from the ethnographic interviews with the informants (Table 15-3). They were: kinds of kids with hair

Table 15-3. Domains of Meaning in the Child's View of Hair Loss

Kinds of kids with hair loss

What hair/head is like

What happens when hair comes out

How to care for hair/head

Thoughts/feelings about hair loss

What others do when hair is falling out

What others should do about hair loss

What to do for others about hair loss

What makes hair loss okay

loss, what hair/head is like during hair loss, what happens when hair comes out, how to care for hair/head, thoughts and feelings about hair loss, what others do when hair is falling out, what others should do about hair loss, what to do for others about hair loss, and what makes hair loss okay.

Labels for the "kinds of kids with hair loss" carried meaning for how children viewed themselves (Table 15-4). For example, "I'm still me," "total withdrawers," "flamboyant," "copers," "super-copers," and "no one knows" suggest categories children use as they refer to the concepts of: being themselves no matter what, withdrawing from it all, being colorful, managing rather well, and

Table 15-4. Domains of Meaning in Kinds of Kids With Hair Loss

I'm still me

Total withdrawers

Flamboyant

Copers

Super-Copers

No one knows

managing the best. Finally, there is the category of "no one knows" to suggest hidden feelings or unwillingness to share.

What hair/head is like during loss differs according to whether the point in time is before chemotherapy, after chemotherapy, after the hair falls out, or after the hair grows back (Table 15-5). Before treatment, we learned the categories children used to describe normal hair (for example: thick, wavy, curly, long). After treatment, children used labels of: thin like spider webs, a huge tangle, big knots, and so on. After hair falls out, the categories were: bald spots, softer, and sticky. After hair comes back, children used categories of: thin, pixielike, baby's hair, and light.

The domain of meaning in what happens when hair comes out gives details on hair coming out in clumps; people pulling at it; activities of brushing, combing, and shaving that make hair come out; and finding hair growing everywhere—in bathtub drains, on pillows and clothing, in coffee, face, nose, mouth, and so on (Table 15-6).

Caring for hair/head suggested many ways of covering, ignoring, accepting, taking care of, and making hair look like it did before the period of hair loss (Table 15-7). Before hair loss, the emphasis appears to be on trying not to disturb it, and after hair loss, on making it look neat.

Thoughts and feelings about hair loss were categorized into those occurring before, during, and after (Table 15-8). Hope, sadness, and anger characterized feelings before hair loss. Missing hair care rituals and how one looks were emphasized after hair loss. The greatest number of ways of thinking and feeling were counted during the hair loss process, from "why me?" to "hate" to "tired of it" to "it's just something that has got to be done." Paranoia, embarrassment, and problems with coverings were also responses.

What others do when hair is falling out portrays how children view their support system (Table 15-9). Nurses and doctors talk, warn, and try to be encouraging. Friends respond in ways conceptualized as "treating me normal," "being embarrassed," "ignoring," "staying away," and "teasing." Some friends tried to hit the new hair just to see how it felt. One teenager lost her friends. Two

Text continues on p. 228.

Table 15-5. Domains of Meaning In What Hair/Head Is Like During Hair Loss

BEFORE TREATMENT	SHOULDER LENGTH
	REAL THICK
	WAVY
	CURLY
	KIND OF LONG
AFTER TREATMENT	SHORT TO VERY SHORT
	THIN TO SORT OF THIN
	MORE SOFT
	LIKE SPIDER WEBS
	COLDER
	YECCHY
	BIG KNOTS
	A HUGE TANGLE
	COMES OFF WHEN TOUCHED
	GROWS MORE
	GROWING BACK
	GROWING DARKER
AFTER HAIR FALLS OUT	STICKY
	BALD SPOTS
	A LOT SOFTER
	COLD
	DARK
	COMFORTABLE
AFTER HAIR COMES BACK	THICK
	BLONDISH
	A LOT
	DARKER
	SOFTER
	PIXIELIKE
	BABY'S HAIR
	LIGHTENED
	LIGHT

Table 15-6. Domains of Meaning In What Happens When Hair Comes Out

WAYS HAIR FALLS OUT	EVERYBODY KEPT PULLING IT
	JUST FALLS OUT
	REAL SLOW
	A LOT
	IN CLUMPS
	A WHOLE BUNCH
	JUST HALF OF IT
	A LITTLE BIT
	TOP PART FIRST AND MOST
WHAT MAKES HAIR COME OUT	BRUSH IT OUT
	WASH IT
	PULL IT OUT
	PULL A BUNCH OUT
	SHAVE IT ALL OFF
	COMB IT OUT
	WIND BLOWS IT OUT
	SCRATCHING AN ITCH
	TOSSING AND TURNING IN BED
	PICKING YOUR HEAD UP IN BED
WHERE HAIR GOES	SETTLES IN BATHTUB DRAIN
	COVERS PILLOW
	PILES ON TABLE
	SHOULDERS
	SHIRT AND EVERYTHING
	COFFEE
	COKE
	HATS
	COUCH
	EVERYWHERE
	FACE
	NOSE
	MOUTH
	EYES

Table 15-7. Domains of Meaning in Caring For Hair/Head

BEFORE HAIR LOSS		ICE TREATMENTS
		TRY NOT TO WASH IT
		DON'T BRUSH IT
		DON'T COMB IT
		NOTICE HAIR CHANGE
		BOTHERED ABOUT LOSING HAIR
DURING HAIR LOSS	COVER	WIGS
		CAPS
		SCARVES
		HATS
	IGNORE	WAIT
		BRUSH
		DON'T TALK ABOUT IT
		MAKE IT LOOK NEAT
	ACCEPT	MAKE 'EM LAUGH
		DON'T WORRY
		TALK TO SELF "NOTHING I CAN DO, SO WAIT"
	TAKE CARE OF HAIR	WASH IT "ANYWAY"
		CUT IT A LITTLE
		BRUSH IT
		COMB IT
		PUT WATER/CALOMEL ON HEAD
	HELP HAIR COME OUT	SHAVE IT
		WASH IT
		SHAMPOO
		COMB
	MAKE IT LOOK LIKE IT DID	
AFTER HAIR LOSS		TRIM IT UP
		MAKE IT LOOK NEAT
		MAKE FUNNY HAIR STYLES

Table 15-8. Domains of Meaning In Thoughts/Feelings About Hair Loss

BEFORE HAIR LOSS	HOPED IT WOULDN'T COME OUT
	SAD AND A LITTLE MAD
DURING HAIR LOSS	ANNOYANCE
	WHY ME?
	DIDN'T LIKE IT
	JUST GOT TIRED OF IT
	NOTHING TO DO BUT WAIT
	DIDN'T WANT TO GO TO SCHOOL
	TERRIBLE
	HATE IT
	JUST SOMETHING THAT'S GOT TO BE DONE
	DON'T TALK ABOUT IT
	GET PARANOID WHEN I'M GOING TO SEE SOMEONE
	TIRED OF PICKING IT UP EVERYWHERE
	LOOKED UGLIER
	BUGGY
	EMBARRASSED
	IMPATIENT
	COVERING HELPS
	SOMETIMES WIGS FIT
	SOMETIMES WIGS DON'T FIT
	SCARVES THAT DON'T SLIP ARE GOOD
AFTER HAIR LOSS	CAN'T DO ANYTHING WITH IT
	I LOOK LIKE A BABY
	MISS WASHING HAIR
	MISS BLOW-DRYING HAIR
	MISS SETTING IT

Table 15-9. Domains of Meaning In What Others Do When Hair Is Falling Out

NURSES/DOCTORS	WARNS ABOUT HAIR LOSS
	TELLS ABOUT HAIR LOSS HAPPENING TO SOME, BUT NOT TO ALL
	SAYS, "THERE'S NOTHING WE CAN DO"
FRIENDS	SAY I LOOK LIKE A BABY
	ACT LIKE SOMETHING IS WRONG
	ACT LIKE IT LOOKS FUNNY
	LOVE ME AS MUCH WITH OR WITHOUT HAIR
	ACT SURPRISED THAT MY HAIR IS REALLY A WIG
	IGNORE IT
	SURPRISED THAT MY HAIR WAS A WIG
	STAY AWAY
	TEASE
	HIT IT TO FEEL HOW IT FEELS
	JUST KIND OF WALK OUT
	DIDN'T LOOK AT FIRST
	LOOKED UP AT SKY
	TREAT ME NORMAL
	TAKE OFF MY HAT
	STARE
FAMILY	FATHER PLAYS WITH HAIR
	MOM TRIMS AND SHAPES HAIR
	SISTER TEASES
	TELL TEASERS TO GO AWAY
	HELP WITH COVERS FOR HEAD
	TREAT ME LIKE THE SAME PERSON

friends were real good friends, however, and remained so. Others were no longer friends when she returned to school after being sick. Family members were generally supportive; however, fathers played tricks and sisters teased. For example, one father knocked on wood to simulate someone at the door. Daughter responded with a rush to don her wig and, subsequently, discovered her father's joke.

"What others should do when hair falls out" illustrates some of the conflict in the experience of hair loss (Table 15-10). "Ignore" is contrasted with "pay

Table 15-10. Domains of Meaning In What Others Should Do When Hair Is Falling Out

IGNORE	TREAT ME LIKE A NORMAL GUY
	TREAT ME THE SAME AS ALWAYS
	TREAT ME LIKE MYSELF
	TREAT ME LIKE A NORMAL PERSON
PAY ATTENTION	LOOK AT ME
	ASK ME ABOUT IT
	TRY TO HELP ME
	HELP ME TO TALK ABOUT IT
	TALK TO MY FACE
INVENT A TREATMENT	TONIC TO PREVENT HAIR LOSS
	MEDICINE TO MAKE HAIR GROW
	ICE CAP
TELL THINGS	EVERYTHING THAT'S GOING TO HAPPEN
	DIFFERENT THINGS HAPPEN TO DIFFERENT PEOPLE

attention," and the role is likely to become "treat me as normal" but "try to help me" and "help me talk about it." "Inventing a new treatment" and "telling things" refer to health professionals and place the burden on them to get rid of the problem, tell what is going to happen, and give hope by suggesting that "I may be different."

The last domains portray philosophic reflections of children in "what to do for others about hair loss" and "what makes hair loss okay" (Tables 15-11 and 15-12). The domains of "staying the same," "ignoring," "teasing and staring," and "being open in communicating" tell us something about the world of all chronically ill children, and what they attempt to do for family, friends, and strangers when they recognize a child's disfigurement; in other words, how chronically ill children care for others. Conceptualizing something acceptable about hair loss suggests a value system in this subculture of childhood in which some things can be seen as funny, or adequately coped with by wearing wigs to disguise baldness or by reassuring oneself that the baldness is not forever.

Table 15-11. Domains of Meaning In What To Do For Others About Hair Loss

BE SAME SELF	
IGNORE	TEASING
	STARING
TALK ABOUT HAIR LOSS	HOW IT HAPPENED
	WHY IT HAPPENED
	WHAT CANCER IS
	WHAT RADIATION IS

Cultural Themes

Whereas domains represent units of cultural knowledge expressed in the language of the informant, cultural themes are different in that they portray a sense of the "whole" of the cultural system and are usually derived from categories of meaning in the language of the ethnographer. Generating themes is a process of invention. The ethnographer analyzes the data to find a unifying principle linking one domain of meaning with another. Four culturally relevant themes emerged from the data:

1. There's nothing to be done.

2. Loss of hair and loss of friends will occur.

3. Get used to it.

4. Treat me as normal.

"There's nothing to be done" portrays the feeling of hopelessness and sense of fatalism that often accompany the hair loss experience in children. Children tell us that there is nothing anyone can do to make the experience easier or less

Table 15-12. Domains of Meaning In What Make Hair Loss Okay

FRIENDS AND FAMILY WHO TREAT ME THE SAME

PEOPLE AT THE HOSPITAL THAT I KNOW

HAVING A WIG

KNOWING ABOUT HOW HAIR GROWS BACK

SAYING FUNNY THINGS ABOUT THE WAY I LOOK

MAKING FUNNY HAIR STYLES

difficult. They say that they must accept the loss, make the best of it, and then wait for their hair to grow back.

A second theme, "loss of hair and loss of friends," speaks of the cruelty in the social world of children, and of the stigma associated with hair loss. Loss of friends follows loss of hair, as though they were equivalent in the world of the child. During the cancer experience, illness, forced absence from school, and hair loss resulted in fewer friends. Friends disappeared because they were uncomfortable around someone without hair. The informants referred to them as "not true friends" and remakred that indeed they kept their "closest friends." A vicious cycle becomes apparent, for as their social world becomes more isolated, children with hair loss become more fearful of going to school and being made fun of, and thus lose more friends. Some children expected their friends to return with the return of their hair. Often what happened was that everyone had new friends except them.

"Get used to it" is similar to a theme found by Berg among the elderly, which she called "working on acceptance.[20] After the initial shock and sense of loss, most children begin to adjust to baldness. Most choose to cover their head with scarves, caps, and wigs to avoid stares and questions, and are thus able to go about daily activities. As long as their family support system thinks it is okay to be bald, the children feel comfortable. Part of "getting use to it" was reflected in joking relationships established between family members and clinic staff. For example, one young boy wore a ski cap in the hottest weather. When people would ask to see his head, his response would be reflexive—he lifted up the front of the cap and returned it to place in one quick motion.

Finally, the theme "treat me as normal" illustrates that children want everyone to know that they have not changed, and they want to believe it themselves. They believe that they are the same person they were before their hair loss. Being accepted as they are is important to them. It just may be that the questions we are asking about body image are grounded in the meanings the child's audience conveys to the child. How "the others" in the world of chronically ill children influence their body image is not a new question.

In summary, this is a brief account of how children view hair loss. If the children were to translate what they have to tell us in the language of professional nursing, which might be conceptualized as rules for self-care, we believe that they might say: (1) Find out more about us; (2) Tell us what is happening; (3) Communicate positive feelings; (4) Teach others how to act toward us; (5) Help us understand that our hair will grow back; and (6) Remember that we are the same, but different. The idea of differences suggests to us that there may be several profiles of kinds of responses to hair loss among children that could be viable for an assessment tool and thereby enhance quality care for children.

REFERENCES

1. Goodenough WH: Cultural anthropology and linguistics. *In* Garvin PL (ed): Report of the Seventh Annual Round Table Meetings of Linguistics and Language Study. Washington, Georgetown University Monograph Series on Languages and Linguistics, No. 9, 1957.
2. Spradley JP: The Ethnographic Interview. New York, Holt, Rinehart and Winston, 1979.
3. Spradley JP: Participant-Observation. New York, Holt, Rinehart, and Winston, 1980.
4. Goodman ME: The Culture of Childhood. New York, Columbia University Press, 1970.
5. Harre R: The conditions for a social psychology of childhood. *In* Richards MPM (ed): Integration of a Child into a Social World. London, Cambridge University Press, 1974, pp 245–262.
6. Aamodt AM: The child's view of health and healing. *In* Batey MV (ed): Communicating Nursing Research, Vol. 5, Boulder, Colorado, Western Council for Higher Education in Nursing, 1962, pp 38–54.
7. Aamodt AM: Social-cultural dimensions of caring in the world of the papago child and adolescent. *In* Leininger M (ed): Transcultural Nursing: Concepts, Theories and Practices. New York, John Wiley & Sons, 1978, pp 37–45.
8. Wagner J: Nursing: The Philosophy and Science of Caring. Boston, Little, Brown and Company, 1979.
9. Leininger M (ed): Transcultural Nursing: Concepts, Theories and Practices. New York, John Wiley & Sons, 1978.
10. Leininger M (ed): Transcultural Nursing: Proceedings from Four Transcultural Nursing Conferences. New York, Masson Publishing Co., 1979.
11. Leininger M: Caring: a central focus of nursing and health care services. Nursing and Health Care 1(3):135–176, 1980.
12. Leininger M: Care: An Essential Human Need. Thorofare, NJ, Charles B. Slack, Inc., 1981.
13. Hyde A: The phenomenon of caring: Part I. Nursing Research Report. American Nurses' Foundation 10(1):1–2, 10–11, 1975.
14. Hyde A: The phenomenon of caring: Parts II, III. Nursing Research Report. American Nurses' Foundation 11:2, 15, 1975.
15. Hyde A: The phenomenon of caring: Part IV. Nursing Research Report. American Nurses' Foundation, 12:2, 1977.
16. Aamodt AM: The care component in health and healing systems. *In* Bauwens E (ed): The Anthropology of Health. St. Louis, C.V. Mosby, 1978, pp 37–45.
17. Aamodt AM: Neighboring: discovering support systems among Norwegian-American women. *In* Messerschmidt DA (ed): Anthropologists at Home in North America: Methods and Issues in the Study of One's own Society. New York, Cambridge University Press, 1981, pp 133–152.
18. Watson J: Nursing: The Philosophy and Science of Caring. Boston, Little, Brown and Company, 1979.
19. Honigmann JJ: Responsibility and nurturance: an Austrian example. J Psychol Anthropol 1(1): 81–100, 1978.
20. Aamodt AM, Berg C: Client-nurse encounters in ambulatory health care settings. Unpublished manuscript, 1979.

16

Caring–The Central Construct for an Associate Degree Nursing Curriculum

HISTORICAL PERSPECTIVE

In October 1979, the Cuesta College nursing faculty received a private donation of $85,000. The gift has allowed the faculty to develop care as the central construct of the associate degree (AD) nursing curriculum. The enriching experience of three years' work is described in this chapter.

Believing, like Leininger, that caring is the central and unifying domain for the body of knowledge and practices of nursing, the faculty sought experts to assist with the task of defining care and the caring subconstructs required to formulate a framework for curriculum development.[1] This effort comprised the first year of the project.

Although some descriptions of care had been offered by philosophers and social scientists such as Gaylin, May, and Mayeroff, no clear definition served adequately to define nursing's understanding of care.[2-4] The faculty struggled to identify the philosophic underpinnings of this precious yet elusive construct. Then the faculty was introduced to the work of Em Olivia Bevis.[5] Bevis had developed a conceptual framework delineating phases of caring from a grounded theory approach.[5] The conceptual framework was applied in the new baccalaureate nursing (BSN) curriculum at Georgia Southern College, Statesboro. After lengthy discussion with Bevis and her colleague, Joyce Murray, it was decided that their philosophy and conceptual framework seemed most suitable to the faculty's perceptions of and beliefs about caring. The caring philosophy and conceptual framework were incorporated into the caring model for the AD nursing curriculum.

THE A.D. "CARING CURRICULUM"

For purposes of brevity, the curriculum components are summarized so that process may be emphasized. It is hoped, however, that the overview will provide a basic understanding regarding how care provides the central curriculum focus. The curriculum is based in humanistic existentialist philosophy. The belief that man is of central importance, has inherent dignity, and is worthy of respect and care simply because he exists, and the basic belief that the most basic and irrefutable freedom is freedom of choice, undergird the philosophic statements and definitions.

Three primary definitions proceed from the philosophy.

1. *Caring*—a feeling of commitment to self and others to the extent that it motivates and energizes action to influence life constructively and positively by increasing intimacy and mutual self-actualization.

2. *Health*—the purpose of all nursing behaviors. Health is determined by the ability of the individual, family, group, or community to set realistic and meaningful goals and to mobilize energy and resources to attain these goals efficiently. This is accomplished while caring about self and others, feeling good about one's self, and helping others feel good about themselves with the fewest possible negative effects on the environment.

3. *Nursing*—a practice discipline that provides a caring service to society directed at prevention of health problems, maintenance of health, care of the sick, restoration to optimal health, and provision of a peaceful death.

THE CONCEPTUAL FRAMEWORK

Components for the conceptual framework were developed by using Waters' model.[6]

Waters refers to Chater's subject category of conceptual framework as a perception of nursing practice, and says that this part of the framework is often referred to as a "nursing practice theory." The latter is a description of how the faculty teaches nursing so that it is practiced in a way that the faculty can practice it. Waters further identifies seven areas that must be addressed in order to provide a picture of the faculty's perception of nursing practice that is clear enough to be implemented in the curriculum, and in classroom and clinical areas. These seven areas are: (1) nursing goals; (2) the problems nurses will see as their domain; (3) the client of the nurse; (4) the nursing behaviors that will be used with the specified clients who have the selected problems; (5) the tools and concepts nurses use in enacting behaviors; (6) the setting in which nurses work with clients; and (7) the work-role relationships nurses establish in order to work with clients toward the goals in the selected settings.

Table 16-1 is presented to demonstrate the effective use of Waters' model. The conceptual elements distinguish how caring is applied within the two levels of nursing education.

Faculties of the associate and baccalaureate degree nursing programs viewed nursing goals, problems, and settings as being similar. The distinctions between practice levels are clients, nursing behaviors, tools and concepts used to enact the nursing behaviors, and work-role relationships. The distinctions may really reflect faculties' efforts to clarify perceptions more than any real differentiation between practice levels. The exceptions, however, were the elements "clients served" and "tools and concepts" used for enacting, in that the Cuesta College nursing faculty did not view the community as an appropriate client for associate degree nursing practice. The Cuesta nursing faculty also held that psychomotor skills are of paramount importance for the nurse prepared through the associate degree program, and these skills were identified as unique caring tools.

DEFINING CURRICULUM OBJECTIVES

In identifying distinctions among nursing levels, Bevis advocated a framework for assessing levels of complexity.[7] These are:

1. The degree of familiarity.

2. The number of variables that must be handled at one time.

3. The amount of structure provided.

4. The degree of intensity in the situation.

5. The level of theory addressed.

The faculty listed all content felt to be requisite to nursing education. Bevis' levels of complexity model was applied first to isolate AD nursing content as perceived by the faculty. Bevis' model was applied again so that an arrangement of AD content from "simple to complex" was designed. After completing this extensive sorting and arranging process, the faculty realized that with few exceptions, the BSN curriculum objectives developed by Bevis and Murray were appropriate for the AD curriculum as well. Ten AD curriculum objectives were designed, and four sets of level objectives were defined. All were arranged according to Bevis' levels of complexity. The curriculum and level objectives appear in Table 16-2.

Text continues on p. 242.

Table 16-1. Comparison of Associate Degree and Baccalaureate Nursing Degree Programs With Waters' Conceptual Elements

Conceptual Elements	Associate Degree Program*	Baccalaureate Nursing Program*
1. Nursing Goals	a. facilitate health b. self-actualization	a. facilitate health b. self-actualization
2. Nursing Problems	a. goal-setting b. energy c. caring	a. goal-setting b. energy c. caring
3. Clients	a. individuals b. families c. groups	a. individuals b. families c. groups d. communities
4. Nursing Behaviors	*Four Categories* a. prevention b. maintenance c. caring d. restoration	*Three Categories* a. protective b. nutritive c. generative
5. Tools/Concepts to Enact Behaviors	a. communication b. teaching/learning c. nursing process d. caring e. energy f. life span g. psychomotor skills	a. communication b. analysis c. management d. teaching/learning *Other Useful Concepts* a. energy b. health c. maturation
6. Settings	a. primary b. secondary c. tertiary	a. primary b. secondary c. tertiary
7. Work-Role Relationships	a. colleagueship b. management c. leadership d. coordination e. advocacy	a. colleagueship b. management c. leadership d. coordination

*The AD Program of the Nursing Division of Cuesta College, San Luis Obispo, and the BSN Program of Georgia Southern College, School of Nursing at Statesboro, Georgia, were used for comparative analysis.

Table 16-2. Curriculum By Behavior Levels Objectives

Upon completion of the Associate Degree Program, the graduate will be able to provide quality nursing care to individuals, families, and groups in a variety of rural and urban settings in a manner acceptable to the diverse population of San Luis Obispo, or similar communities, by

Curriculum Objective #1
Utilizing nursing concepts to facilitate health and self-actualization by solving goal-setting, energy, and caring problems.

LEVEL I	*LEVEL II*	*LEVEL III*	*LEVEL IV*
At the end of Level I, the student will be able to:	At the end of Level II, the student will be able to:	At the end of Level III, the student will be able to:	At the end of Level IV, the student will be able to:
Interpret nursing concepts that provide a structure for nursing practice.	Use selected nursing concepts to facilitate health and self-actualization by solving specific goal-setting, energy, and caring problems.	Utilize nursing concepts to facilitate health by achieving selected goals which relate to families.	Implement and evaluate nursing concepts to facilitate health and self-actualization by solving complex goal-setting, energy, and caring problems.

Curriculum Objective #2
Using a data base from the humanities and sciences to support nursing activities.

LEVEL I	*LEVEL II*	*LEVEL III*	*LEVEL IV*
Support nursing activities with concepts from the humanities and sciences.	Apply decision-making data derived from the humanities and sciences to support nursing activities.	Explain rationale to support nursing activities for families that is drawn from concepts from humanities and sciences.	Integrate rationale for nursing activities that is drawn from concepts from humanities and sciences.

(Continued)

Table 16-2. (Continued)

Curriculum Objective #3
Using the concept of caring as a basis for providing nursing care, implementing the behaviors of prevention, maintenance, care, and restoration.

LEVEL I	*LEVEL II*	*LEVEL III*	*LEVEL IV*
Use the caring process as a basis for providing nursing care, implementing the behaviors of prevention, maintenance, care, and restoration in highly structured situations with the individual client.	Use the concept of caring as a basis for providing nursing care, implementing the behaviors of prevention, maintenance, care, and restoration in moderately structured situations.	Demonstrate the caring process for providing care to families, implementing the behaviors of prevention, maintenance, care, and restoration in moderately structured situations.	Use the concept of caring as a basis for providing nursing care in implementing the behaviors of prevention, maintenance, care, and restoration in minimally structured situations.

Curriculum Objective #4
Being responsible and accountable for self and one's nursing practice.

LEVEL I	*LEVEL II*	*LEVEL III*	*LEVEL IV*
Discuss the factors involved in being responsible and accountable for self and one's nursing practice.	Make choices about personal behaviors that influence accountability for self and one's nursing practice.	Demonstrate personal behaviors that influence accountability for self and one's nursing practice.	Evaluate personal behaviors that influence accountability for self and one's nursing practice.

(Continued)

Table 16-2. *(Continued)*

Curriculum Objective #5
Providing nursing care to clients of diverse cultures utilizing the tools of communication, teaching, nursing process, caring, energy, and psychomotor skills.

LEVEL I	*LEVEL II*	*LEVEL III*	*LEVEL IV*
Provide nursing care to individual adults of diverse cultures utilizing the tools of communication, teaching, nursing process, caring, energy, and psychomotor skills in highly structured situations.	Provide nursing care throughout the life span for selected clients of diverse cultures utilizing the tools of communication, teaching, nursing process, caring, energy, and psychomotor skills in moderately structured situations.	Provide nursing care for selected families of diverse cultures utilizing the tools of teaching, communication, nursing process, caring, energy, and psychomotor skills in moderately structured situations.	Provide nursing care for selected high-risk families of diverse cultures utilizing the tools of communication, teaching, nursing process, caring, energy and psychomotor skills in minimally structured situations.

Curriculum Objective #6
Using research findings in nursing practice.

LEVEL I	*LEVEL II*	*LEVEL III*	*LEVEL IV*
Read nursing research articles.	Use research findings in selected client settings.	Use selected nursing research findings for their applicability to nursing care of families.	Use research findings in diverse client situations.

(Continued)

Table 16-2. *(Continued)*

	LEVEL I	LEVEL II	LEVEL III	LEVEL IV
Curriculum Objective #7 Establishing learning patterns that will provide the means for life-long personal and professional growth.	Express own learning needs based on personal and professional growth awareness.	Demonstrate an accountability for own personal and professional learning.	Demonstrate behavior that facilitates personal and professional growth.	Evaluate personal and professional growth.
Curriculum Objective #8 Developing work-role relationships with other members of the health team.	Identify work-role relationships among members of the health team.	Communicate with members of the health team based on knowledge of the skills which contribute to work-role relationships.	Plan with other members of the health team.	Evaluate work-role relationships with other members of the health team.
	Describe the behaviors of nurse advocacy based on the analysis of the factors involved in advocacy.	Demonstrate the behaviors of nurse advocacy based on the analysis of the factors involved in advocacy.	Demonstrate the behaviors of nurse advocacy in providing nursing care for families.	Apply the nursing process to the role of nurse advocate.

(Continued)

Table 16-2. *(Continued)*

Curriculum Objective #9
Practicing nursing that is responsive to current and changing community health care needs.

LEVEL I	*LEVEL II*	*LEVEL III*	*LEVEL IV*
Identify community health resources.	Begin to use community health resources to meet health needs of selected clients.	Utilize available community health resources in caring for families.	Evaluate response of community health resources to community health needs.

Curriculum Objective #10
Enacting the role of leader in nursing practice and as a member of the community.

LEVEL I	*LEVEL II*	*LEVEL III*	*LEVEL IV*
Describe the behaviors necessary to being a caring colleague.	Demonstrate behavior necessary to being a caring colleague and a caring nurse.	Apply the caring component to the nursing leadership role.	Practice caring leadership skills by organizing nursing care, participating in professional organizations, and through community involvement.

COMPARISON OF ASSOCIATE AND BACCALAUREATE NURSING CURRICULUM OBJECTIVES

A comparison of curriculum objectives between the associate and baccalaureate nursing programs is found in Table 16–3. From this table, one will note that each program has ten identical curriculum objectives, with distinctions identifiable as level objectives. The differences between the two programs appear to be related to the levels of complexity, as described by Bevis. For example, in an analysis of Curriculum Objective #5, there are specific descriptive terms used in the baccalaureate nursing program—"tools of communication, analysis, management, and teaching/learning"—whereas in the associate degree program, the descriptive statement is "tools of communication, teaching/learning, nursing process, caring, energy, and psychomotor skills." The distinguishing factors, however, are primarily the faculty's expectations for students, described by the specific level objectives. For example, the faculty of the baccalaureate nursing program expects students in Level I to "provide care for *selected clients*— utilizing tools of communication and analysis." The faculty of the associate degree program expects students to experience or handle more structure with less intensity and to use a simple level of theory. The associate degree nursing faculty expects students to "provide care to *individual adults*—in *highly structured* situations." Level IV objectives for the associate degree program require students to "provide nursing care for *selected* high-risk families (specific small groups) and in minimally structured situations." This expectation is comparable to the lower-level baccalaureate program expectation of Level II: namely, to "provide nursing care for *selected clients . . .*" These comparative examples seem to represent most of the level objectives identified by the faculties of the associate and baccalaureate nursing programs.

While there is some overlapping in the level objective expectations between the two curricula, the objectives distinguish two levels of nursing practice based upon and centered on caring. Bevis' levels of complexity allowed an arrangement of content that flows logically throughout the associate degree program and continues into the baccalaureate program. Basic caring content is introduced at the associate degree level and defines that level of practice. Caring content has been advanced and structured for baccalaureate nursing practice. Throughout both curricula, caring was used as the overriding conceptual construct.

Table 16-3. Selected Examples of Associate and Baccalaureate Curricula Level Objectives

Objectives	Associate Degree Nursing Program	Baccalaureate Nursing Program
Curriculum	#1 Utilizing nursing *concepts* to facilitate health and self-actualization by solving goal-setting, energy, and caring problems	#1 Utilizing nursing *theory* to facilitate health and self-actualization by solving goal-setting, energy, and caring problems
Level	I *Interpret* nursing concepts.	I *Identify selected* nursing theory. Utilize *simple* baseline assessments for classifying.
	II *Use selected* nursing concepts—by solving *specific* problems.	II *Use selected* nursing theories—by solving *specific* problems.
	III *Utilize* nursing concepts to facilitate health by achieving *selected* goals which relate to *families*.	III *Utilize* nursing theory—by solving *complex* problems.
	IV *Implement and evaluate* nursing concepts—by solving *complex* problems.	
Curriculum	#3 Using the concept of caring as a basis for providing nursing care, implementing the behaviors of prevention, maintenance, care, and restoration.	#3 Using the concepts of caring as a basis for providing nursing care, implementing the behaviors of protection, surveillance, curative, and generativity.
Level	I *Uses the caring process* as a basis for providing nursing care, implementing the behaviors of *prevention, maintenance, care, and restoration* in *highly structured* situations with *individual clients*.	I *Uses the caring process* as a basis for providing nursing care, implementing behaviors of *protection, surveillance, and nurture* in *highly structured* situations.
	II *—moderately structured* situations.	II *Uses the concept of caring—* implementing the behaviors of protection, surveillance, nurture, *curative, and generativity in complex* situations.

(Continued)

Table 16-3. (Continued)

Objectives	Associate Degree Nursing Program	Baccalaureate Nursing Program
	III *Demonstrates* the caring process for providing care to *families*—in *moderately structured* situations.	III *Uses* the caring process—*based on the analysis of factors influencing caring.*
	IV *Uses the concept* of caring as a basis—in *minimally structured* situations.	
Curriculum	#5 Providing nursing care to clients of diverse cultures, utilizing the tools of communication, teaching, nursing process, caring, energy, and psychomotor skills.	#5 Provides nursing care to clients of diverse cultures, utilizing the tools of communication, analysis, management, and teaching/learning.
Level	I *Provides nursing care to individual adults* utilizing the tools— in *highly structured* situations.	I *Provide care to selected clients* of diverse cultures—based on *protective, surveillance, and nutrative skills.*
	II *Provides nursing care throughout the life span*—in *moderately structured* situations.	II *Provide* nursing care for *selected clients*—communication, analysis, *management, and teaching/learning.*
	III *Provides nursing care for selected families*—in *moderately structured* situations.	III *Manage* nursing care of clients utilizing the tools.
	IV *Provides nursing care for selected high-risk clients*—in *minimally structured* situations.	

THE CURRICULUM DESIGN

The curriculum plan included 14 courses arranged into a four-semester program, as seen in Table 16–4.

Basically, the design introduces caring as the overriding conceptual construct. Philosophy, conceptual framework, and definitions are major focuses of the first-level courses. Since the Cuesta faculty believes that self-care is inseparable from care for others, students learn self-care theory and are expected to use these techniques not only in their nursing practice but also throughout the nursing education program. Caring concepts and behaviors are introduced and expanded with increasing depth as the student progresses through the curriculum.[1] Practicum courses allow development of caring tools. Complexity of care increases and settings change until, upon completion of the curriculum, the graduate is expected to apply the caring process in nursing individuals, families, and selected groups in structured and some unstructured settings. Throughout, emphasis is on wellness and the unique meaning that concept holds for a culturally diverse community. With that in mind, a course was designed in the third level to present alternate health care modalities. The curriculum design plans for the unique needs of licensed vocational nurses and others with nursing background so that equivalency credit is granted. However, all graduates are required to complete the two foundational courses: Introduction to Caring and Professional Self-Care. Course outlines were developed. The curriculum was sanctioned by the college curriculum committee, and, with much praise, by the California State Board of Registered Nursing.

THE CURRICULUM IMPLEMENTED

After a full year of implementation, it is difficult for the architects of the program to restrain enthusiasm. The results so far are encouraging and rewarding. It is a hard task to summarize the many outcomes.

Early in the change process, it was recognized that faculty education was essential. In addition to curriculum workshops, faculty participated in total in a variety of endeavors that prepared them for the responsibility of introducing the new curriculum. Although input from consultants was significant, it was the faculty who functioned as the curriculum architects, and it would be the faculty who would implement the curriculum. The faculty fully accepted this part of their responsibility. For example, in addition to five three-day intensive curriculum retreats and weekly faculty meetings, faculty have conducted research and innovative projects related to caring. Two faculty members have completed doctoral programs, and their dissertations related to aspects of caring.

The faculty believed that teaching and learning strategies must reflect caring. Therefore, students are considered partners in the learning process. A system of facilitator-assisted learning formalizes this belief. After an intensive two-day

Table 16-4. Cuesta College Curriculum For Associate Degree in Nursing

Semester One	Semester Two	Level One	Level Two	Level Three	Level Four
*Chemistry 10–Introductory Chemistry (4 units)	Microbiology 1–General Bacteriology (4 units)	Nursing 1–Nurse Caring (2 units)			
Zoology 5–Human Anatomy (4 units)	Zoology 6–General Physiology (5 units)	**Nursing 1A–Nurse Caring Concepts I (3 units)	**Nursing 2A–Nurse Caring Concepts II (3 units)	Nursing 3A–Nurse Caring of Families—Concepts (4 units)	Nursing 4A–Nurse Caring for People at Risk—Concepts (3 units)
		**Nursing 1B–Nurse Caring Tools I (5 units)	**Nursing 2B–Nurse Caring Tools II (7 units)	Nursing 3B–Nurse Caring of Families—Tools (4 units)	Nursing 4B–Nurse Caring for People at Risk—Tools (5 units)
		Nursing 1C—Professional Self-Care (2 units)	**Nursing 2D—Decision-Making Data I (3 units)	Nursing 3D—Decision-Making Data II (3 units)	Nursing 4C—Professional Care of Self and Others (3 units)
		Psychology 1A—Introductory Psychology (3 units)	Sociology 1A—Introductory Sociology (3 units)	Nursing 3E—Alternate Health Care Modalities (2 units)	
		English 1A—Introductory English (3 units)	History requirement (3 units)	Humanities (3 units)	
				Speech 1A—Introductory Speech (3 units)	

*Not required if high school chemistry is completed.
**Not required if Licensed Vocational Nurses.

workshop, selected students serve as "facilitators" among small groups of their peers. Thus far, it seems that facilitator-assisted learning is an exceptional method which humanizes nursing education.

Strategies that promote active learning are incorporated to accommodate the wide variety of learning needs. Students are a heterogeneous group, with the differing age, sex, social, and cultural backgrounds and academic preparations typical of AD students. Students quickly form support networks, which foster nurse-nurse caring.

A sophisticated caring tools laboratory was developed so that tools can be practiced in simulated learning experiences. The tools lab allows students to develop confidence and competence in practicing caring skills — a prerequisite to caring nursing practice. Competency-based testing assures both faculty and students of safe practice prior to clinical application.

Students are respected as mature adult learners. Representatives enthusiastically share concerns at regular faculty meetings as well as offering helpful ideas for positive change.

Experience thus far shows that students struggle with the caring framework in the first level. Some even protest and misinterpret, particularly those who are rigidly biased against humanistic-existentialist philosophy. Caring content touches deep personal value systems. Therefore, students require additional support and understanding at this time. However, by level two most students have internalized the caring framework and are using it to organize their nursing care. Students are then ready to discuss their personal caring behaviors and separate those from other noncaring feelings and processes such as rescuing, overidentifying, concern, and sexuality (which formerly they understood to be "caring" feelings and behaviors). Additionally, they more readily recognize caring and noncaring behaviors of staff in the practice setting. Most encouraging is that students recognize (and protest) when faculty do not adhere to the caring framework with teacher-mode tests.

Overall, comments from the community, the students, and the faculty have been positive. Morale has remained high, and a deep commitment to developing caring as the central construct of nursing education and practice is plainly evident.

CAUTION

Caring is essential to nursing. Moreover, caring may be the unique domain of nursing, distinguishing it from all other disciplines. As Leininger so aptly stated: "Caring is the essence of nursing and the unique and unifying focus of the profession."[1] The renaissance of care as a vital new direction for nursing has renewed the vigor of nurse researchers, practitioners, scientists, and educators. It would be appealing for curriculum architects to design other curricula based on caring. Such a move is premature.

Caring as the central curriculum construct needs careful research and refinement. Further research is essential to sort out this obscure concept more clearly. The caring model as presented requires validity. A wealth of data will surface through the experience of the two existing programs. These data, together with those gleaned from ongoing caring research, will provide the critical ingredients for a clearer theory of caring. Established as an all-encompassing theory base, caring would then provide the central construct for curriculum design and nursing practice. Thereby, the unique societal contribution of nursing would be distinguished.

It is to this endeavor that a committed team of researchers, scientists, practitioners, and educators, energized by caring, dedicates its effort.

REFERENCES

1. Leininger MM (ed): Caring: An Essential Human Need. Thorofare, NJ, Charles B. Slack, Inc.,1981, p 3.
2. Gaylin W: Caring. New York, Alfred A. Knopf, 1976.
3. May R: Love & Will. New York, W.W. Norton & Co., 1969.
4. Mayeroff M: On Caring. New York, Harper & Row, 1971.
5. Bevis EO: Conceptual framework: The knowledge component. In Bevis EO: Curriculum Building in Nursing: A Process. St. Louis, MO, C.V. Mosby & Co., 1978, pp 110-122.
6. Waters V: Conceptual Framework Workshop, Calgary, Alberta, Canada, 1976.
7. Bevis EO: Curriculum Workshop with Cuesta College Nursing Faculty, San Luis Obispo, CA, 1980.

17

Client Care-Seeking Behaviors and Nursing Care

INTRODUCTION

This study is focused on client care-seeking behaviors and the client's response to nursing care. Utilizing a grounded theory approach, 35 interviews were studied for common characteristics. Three questions emerged from the preliminary readings: (1) Why do clients seek care? (2) What do they expect when they seek care? (3) What are the outcomes from their point of view? The initial perusal of the data provided the research questions and the impetus for this study.

PURPOSES OF THE STUDY

The purposes of the study were to: (1) identify the characteristics and processes inherent in client care-seeking behavior in a community health setting; and (2) identify the sources of client satisfaction and dissatisfaction with the process of receiving nursing care.

DEFINITIONS

Category: A class or dimension in a scheme of classification.
Characteristic: A distinguishing trait or property.
Phase: A sequence in a series of related events.
Stage: Related segments that together make up a phase.
Dimension: The range or degree over which a particular characteristic extends.
Interaction: Mutual or reciprocal action between at least two people.

Activity: A generalized behavior utilized by the nurse as a response to client need, eg, support.

Action: A specific act utilized by the nurse that constitutes one element of an activity, eg, listening.

Self-referred: Clients who made the initial contact with the workshop themselves.

Other-referred: Clients whose contact with the agency was made by other persons on their behalf.

Care: The provision of assistance, support, or other facilitative acts toward or for another individual.[1]

Caring: A process that allows the client to grow and self-actualize himself/herself.

DESIGN AND PROCEDURES

The study was exploratory in nature. The researcher who conducted the analysis had not been involved in the interviews. The transcripts of interviews from a data bank formed the unit of analysis. A grounded theory approach, using a constant comparative method of analysis, was used to generate categories. Utilizing the categories, a model of care-seeking was constructed.

POPULATION AND DATA COLLECTION

The population consisted of 35 clients who had visited a community agency, "The Health Workshop," a facility staffed entirely by nurses. The clients were observed as they visited with a nurse and were then interviewed by one of two interviewers between May 2 and August 25, 1978. Eight nurses were involved in the client visits. One nurse was observed with only one client; one nurse was observed with nine clients; while the mode (three nurses) was five clients. All client interviewers were adult, and usually only one member of the family took part in the interviews.

The number of visits that clients had made to nurses at the time of the observed visit ranged from one to 100, with a mode of four. In 17 cases, the identified problem centered on a female, in 3 on a male, and in 15 cases more than one member of a family was involved. Fifteen clients had been visited in their own homes and 20 in the workshop. Twenty-seven clients were self-referred, and eight were referred from other agencies.

LIMITATIONS OF THE STUDY

1. The constraints prevented construct validation of the characteristics.

2. Negative findings in some small subgroups were only partially explained due to the small numbers of cases involved.

3. Data were precollected so that weak areas could not be supplemented by the addition of more cases.

4. Problem dimensions were not mutually exclusive, based on the results of the reliability check.

ANALYSIS OF THE DATA

The constant comparative method used to examine the data employs joint coding and analysis to generate theory. Such theory is integrated, consistent, plausible, close to the data, and in a form clear enough to be readily, if only partially, operationalized for testing in quantitative research.[2,3]

In conducting the analysis, the first step was to read all the interviews to identify broad categories in the data. Once tentative categories were identified, interviews were reanalyzed, and the categories were examined for common characteristics. The interviews were examined in sets of five. After the second set of five interviews was analyzed, they were compared with the first set of five, and the categories and characteristics were revised as necessary. Subsequently, each batch of interviews was compared with the initial batch. Exceptions were noted, and reasons for the differences were examined. The data were then examined for processes related to the characteristics. The next stage was reexamination of the categories, characteristics, and processes in an attempt to delimit the theory.

Validity of categories, the types of problems, and the types of care were established by a panel of judges. The properties and relationships were not validated by the panel due to time constraints related to their workload and the deadline for completion of the study. Reliability of the categories was established between coders. The quality of the interviews varied. While there was consistency in the information obtained by the two interviewers, in later interviews fewer probe questions were used. For the purpose of this analysis, the data were less rich than in earlier interviews.

CARING AND CARE-SEEKING

Care is generally accepted as one of the attributes central to nursing. Leininger defined care and caring in terms of assistive, supportive, or facilitative acts toward or for another individual.[1] Caring thus involves a helping relationship between the nurse and another. Mayeroff sees caring as a process that helps another grow and self-actualize himself or herself.[4] This suggests that caring is a developmental process which takes place in a supportive environment. Care-seeking can be differentiated from cure-seeking in that in the latter case, the patients/clients see themselves as having medical symptoms that need curing, whereas in care-seeking the clients see themselves in a vulnerable position due to some form of life stress. They need comfort, concern, love, and nurturing from another person, along with support and guidance, to enable them to resume their former coping behaviors. In this study, the majority of clients came to the Workshop seeking means of improving their health or their families' health. They did not come expecting an illness to be cured. There were two clients who saw themselves as "ill," but they came only to seek information on where to go to be cured because they were unfamiliar with facilities in the area. It can thus be argued that the process the clients were involved in was one of care-seeking, in that they looked for nursing actions that were assistive, facilitative, or supportive in helping them to resolve their problems or move toward their goals.[1] The ways in which the clients identified a need for care, the means of seeking care, and the consequences of care were identified in the data analysis.

PHASES OF CARE-SEEKING

Three definite phases of care-seeking were identified: a preactive, an interactive, and a postactive phase. These phases formed the framework for the analysis. The dimensions, the behaviors, and the activities relating to each phase were examined, and the processes of care-seeking were identified (Fig. 17-1).

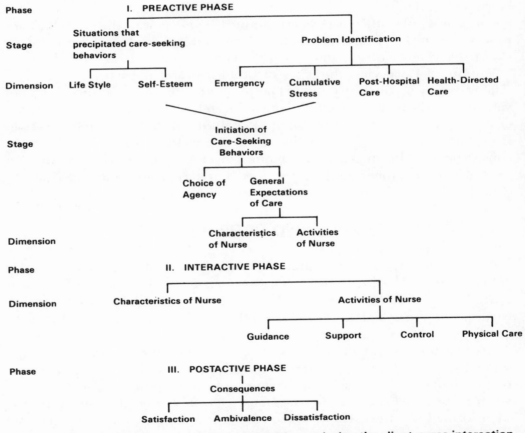

Figure 17-1. The model of care-seeking utilized for analyzing the client-nurse interaction.

Preactive Phase

The preactive phase consisted of three stages: (1) a situation that precipitated care-seeking behavior: (2) the identification of a problem by the client; and (3) the initiation of care-seeking behaviors

Stage 1: Factors that Precipitated Care-Seeking Behavior. Among self-referred clients, a preactive phase occurred before contact was made with the Workshop. Some common dimensions were identified related to the interaction of factors in the clients' lifestyles with their self-esteem. Self-esteem was used to denote the ways in which the client viewed his own capabilities and body image. Lifestyle was a factor in the environment that affected the individual as he went about his daily activities.

Table 17-1 demonstrates some of the lifestyle and self-esteem factors that made the clients identify a need for care. Some clients already had stresses and strains in their life, while others sought care because they wanted to prevent problems by improving their lifestyle; for example, a "good mother" produces a "healthy baby."

Table 17-1. Preactive Phase: Situations That Precipitated Care-Seeking Behaviors

Situation	Threat to Lifestyle	Effect on Self-Esteem
Chronic Pain	Malfunctioning support system	Psychologic threat to self image
Discharge after hospitalization	Unstable support system	Dependence & independence
		Threat to self as independent individual
Divorce, move to new area	No support system	Threat to psychologic and social image
Chronic obesity	Social consequences	Threat to body image
Negative experience with previous health care	Robbed of independence	Feeling of helplessness

From the data, the following processes related to care-seeking emerged:

1. When factors in the individual's lifestyle exerted so much force on the individual's self-esteem that he perceived himself as being unable to resolve his problem without aid, care-seeking behavior was initiated.

2. When an individual perceived that a change in lifestyle would be beneficial to his health but did not believe that he had adequate resources to create this change, care-seeking behavior was initiated.

Stage 2: Problem Identification. The dimensions of the problems presented by the clients were limited to four major categories: emergencies; cumulative stress; posthospital (self-referred), and health promotion.

Emergencies were situations in which the clients perceived that their problems required immediate input, and in which the purpose of seeking care was to get attention at that time and at that time only. *Cumulative stress* was identified when clients presented with evidence of multiple problems or one problem that had built up over time. *Posthospital care* was the term used to identify those clients who referred themselves following discharge from the hospital. Generally, these clients found that they had difficulty accepting independence and responsibility for themselves following a period of dependence. *Health promotion* was the term used to identify clients who came to the Workshop seeking health measures that would change their lifestyle. They could be seeking to decrease the effect of chronic disease (diabetes, asthma) or might be looking toward a new direction in their life (pregnancy, family planning). The client might also be seeking measures to decrease illness potential (weight reduction).

Processes involved in problem identification (and presentation) were:

1. Having perceived a need for help, the individual identified a problem or goal with which to approach a health care agent or agency.

2. A dominant problem was selected, but the presenting problem might be only one symptom of a more complex situation.

3. Clients who went through an interagency or interagent referral process might not have an identified problem or goal.

Stage 3: Initiation of Care-Seeking Behaviors. After a client had identified a problem, care-seeking behavior began. Care-seeking behavior involved both identification of an agency or agent able to provide help in the solution of an identified problem or goal and the development of an expectation of care. For some clients, expediency was an important dimension of care-seeking. They looked for a facility that was close to home and where they would receive prompt service. All clients classified as emergencies were concerned with expediency. Similar behavior was identified by Ingram, who found that in an emergency, clients utilized the nearest service whether or not the facility was appropriate.[5]

The role of a stimulus in directing a client's attention to a service once a problem had been identified appeared to be another important dimension of care-seeking. Friends and neighbors provided information, as did nurses who spoke to groups. Friends' information was sometimes gained from attendance at an "Open House" at the Workshop. Verbal stimuli appeared to be most important; however, clients frequently gained additional information from brochures and advertisements after their attention had been focused on the Workshop as an available service.

A third dimension of care-seeking was the client's previous experience with health care agencies. Several clients who came to the Workshop were looking for an alternate service because they felt that they were not receiving adequate help from health care agents or agencies with whom they were already involved. These clients expressed negative feelings about previous contacts with the health care system.

General Expectations of Care. Interactions were apparent between problem identification, selection of an agency, and the development of an expectation of care. In reality, these are interdependent activities rather than separated in time. It was also apparent that clients did approach the agency with an expectation of the care they would receive and of the personality and characteristics of the individual who would give that care.

Clients frequently made contact with the Workshop because they sought increased knowledge about a self-identified problem or condition. However, clients saw themselves as able to manage their own problems so long as they received needed information and support from a nurse. The nurse was expected to be sympathetic to their problems. The expected prototype of this nurse, for most clients, appeared to be a knowledgeable individual, skilled in giving care, who would be reliable and respect confidentiality.

Three major activities that clients expected the nurse to perform were physical care, support, and guidance. Clients who identified their own primary problem as a need for help with physical care also expected support and guidance if they were self-referred. However, clients who were referred by hospital personnel either were unable to define expectations or did not identify support and guidance as nursing activities. The nursing actions identified by clients as providing support included listening and reassurance. Reassurance included reinforcement of the client's own observations and decisions. The most important nursing action in relation to guidance was provision of information. Expected nursing actions related to physical care were weighing, taking blood pressure, taking a pulse, bathing, and wound dressing.

A small group of clients (seven) who showed a lack of external control in their own lifestyle expected the nurse to act in an authoritarian manner and to impose controls within which they would have to function. This group showed a parallel between their lack of self control in lifestyle behavior and their expectation that the nurse would set limits for them.

In summary, the expected processes in relation to nursing intervention were:

1. Through the use of support, the nurse would reduce the client's anxiety and tension so that he would be able to resume control of his own affairs.

2. Through the use of guidance, the nurse would enable the client to resume his own problem-solving or to make progress toward his health goals.

3. Clients who lacked internal control in their lifestyle expected external control when seeking health care.

The Interactive Phase

The second phase, designated as the interactive phase in this study, consisted of the clients' perceptions of their visit with a nurse. In the interview, clients described their perception of the characteristics and behavior of the nurse during the interaction. In most instances, clients described nursing activities that were related to guidance and support, which were also the behaviors most commonly expected by the clients when they sought help. Clients described the nurse as knowledgeable, caring, gentle, skilled, reliable, concerned, and easy to talk to, putting one at ease. The nurse was viewed as having time to listen and as accepting the client's problem even when he was afraid that it might be viewed as trivial.

Supportive activities were those that sustained clients in their endeavors so that they were more likely to succeed in solving their problem or reaching their perceived goal. Guidance activities were those activities that provided direction for individuals in selecting their own course of action. The activities described included sharing information, acting as a sounding board for the client's ideas, and providing alternative resources when the client lacked information. The nurse was perceived as helping clients make their own decisions and not as making decisions for them.

Among the clients referred by other agencies or agents, there was a small group who did not identify a need for guidance and support. While they described actions related to such activities, they did not see them as relevant to their needs. When physical care was given by the nurses, the activities involved were congruent with the expectations of the clients. The clients who were referred from a hospital and who had no clear expectations of care suffered role confusion when physical care was not provided by the nurse.

Processes involved in the client-nurse interaction were the following.

1. Provision of supportive activities resulted in reduction of tension, enabling clients to resume some or all of their normal coping behaviors.

2. Provision of guidance allowed the clients to select a course of action and to move toward the solution of problems or the establishment of new goals.

3. The provision of guidance and support to families whose problems were of a long-term nature resulted in a sense of security, which appeared to be related to the perception that they had acquired a functional support system.

4. Clients who did not have a clearly defined goal or purpose did not see nursing activities as relevant even when they addressed the problem identified by the referring agency.

The Postactive Phase: Consequences of Care-Seeking

In the postactive phase, the clients looked back on the interaction with a nurse and assessed feelings of satisfaction, dissatisfaction, or ambivalence with the process.

Clients who were satisfied either: (1) saw a resolution of the problems, (2) had identified new goals, (3) perceived their tension to be reduced so that they could independently resume problem-solving, or (4) perceived that they were making progress toward their goals.

Ambivalence or dissatisfaction were present: (1) if the client's expectation of care did not coincide with his perception of the care given, and (2) if the client did not perceive the care as necessary, that is, if he had no identified problem and generally no expectations of the care that he needed from a nurse.

Client Satisfaction with Nursing Care. Clients who expressed satisfaction with their care identified some common elements in describing the reason for their response. These included reduction of tension (reassurance and relief were terms used by clients); finding someone who would listen to them; and finding someone who could provide them with information, enabling them to understand or solve their own problems.

While some clients identified progress in resolving their presenting problems, others expressed satisfaction if they perceived that the nursing interaction provided support, even if progress toward solving their problem was not achieved. For example, one client whose husband had had a stroke realized that he would not recover and that her goal for him was not feasible, but she did show a positive response to the nurse's visit, since she felt that someone was sharing her responsibilities with her.

Even when the nurse did not identify one particular client's covert problem—her fear of battering her child—when the nurse behaved in a way congruent with the client's expectations, the outcome was satisfactory from the client's viewpoint. In this instance, the nurse had listened to the concern about her son's temper tantrums and had given advice on child behavior. This client had perceived her need as having someone to listen to her and give advice, and she felt that the nurse had met this need.

Ambivalence or Dissatisfaction with Nursing Care. Out of 35 clients, seven were ambivalent or dissatisfied with nursing care. These clients came from two groups: (1) those whose primary goal was weight reduction, and (2) those who were referred from other agencies. The mechanisms that created a lack of satisfaction appeared to differ between the two groups.

Seven clients contacted the clinic with a primary goal of weight reduction. Of these, four were satisfied with their care, two were ambivalent, and one was clearly dissatisfied. The nurse's action in each case was clearly related to the goal. However, in looking at the client's expectation of nursing action and the perceived action of the nurse in the situation, there was a lack of congruence between expected and perceived actions in the case of the three who were not satisfied with their care.

There were eight clients referred from other agencies. Of these, four did not understand the reason for their referral, and they did not have a clearly identified purpose for seeing the nurse or a clear expectation of her role. These four were all ambivalent about the care given.

Processes involved in consequences of care-seeking were:

1. When the client perceived progress toward solution of a problem or achievement of a goal, satisfaction with the interaction ensued.

2. When expectations were not congruent with the perceived interaction, ambivalence or dissatisfaction with care resulted.

3. When a client had not defined a problem or had no expectations of care, the result was ambivalence or dissatisfaction with the intervention.

The following case study illustrates the process the client undertakes in order to seek and receive care.

CASE STUDY

Mrs. KK had a five-year-old son who had repeated attacks of bronchitis and was diagnosed as having allergic problems. The source of his allergies was unknown.

She identified her need for help in the following way:

> You go through a period when it's all right, then you get hit with a bad season again . . . each time it gets a little more frustrating. I think sometimes you need more than just somebody giving a penicillin prescription constantly for a child with bronchitis; if you could prevent the bronchitis by any other means then that's ideal.

> Just because you're a mother doesn't automatically mean you know all that stuff about your kids.

Mrs. KK identified her goal in the following words:

> I want to know how to deal with a child with allergies, what to do to help alleviate them.

This goal was classed as health-related, since she had previously expressed her desire to prevent the recurrent bronchitis, if possible, so that the need for treatment with antibiotics would be reduced. Recurrent infection because of allergies, and the development of ways to manage the situation to reduce illness, were identified as the major problems by the mother.

Mrs. KK contacted the Workshop because she had seen an advertisement in the local paper and believed a service to be available.

> I thought they had advertised, "Come and see the nurses about allergy problems!" So I did; it seemed the best thing to do. I heard they had a library . . . books on allergies and food allergies, that's really why I went to see them.

Mrs. KK expected to be able to talk with a nurse and thought that the nurse would be able to help her by providing information.

> I felt that there's somebody you could talk to about your problem. She could give you information. It's frustrating when you have no one to talk to.

Mrs. KK described her interaction with the nurse as follows:

> When I went the first time I took a couple of books out . . . She (the nurse) said if I came in with him (the child) she would show me how to drain the bronchial tubes in the mornings, which has helped him, and she suggested I get a cool vaporizer for the night-time.

> We talked generally about how he reacts to things . . . that bother me . . . how he was reacting now the hay fever season was starting . . . We talked about the allergy clinic . . . she gave me two names to call.

> She suggested that I try making a record of what foods were being eaten so then I could see what had been eaten in the past 48 hours or so.

The nurse here utilized guidance, provided the mother with new information, and helped her develop new skills. The mother was shown how to collect data to help identify possible allergies. The nurse acted in a way consistent with expectations.

The client viewed the nurse as "particularly nice, particularly helpful" and added that she found the nurse to be knowledgeable.

> I feel I have something positive now instead of just waiting until it happens again and running off to the doctor. I think the nurse has helped me cope with him a little better . . . I understand it better and I understand the mechanism of the lung. I would certainly recommend the Workshop to (other) people.

PROPOSITIONS

Based on the findings of this study, five tentative propositions relating to nursing intervention were formulated. These can be tested in future studies. Validation in a variety of settings, both hospital and community, would support or rule out their generalizability.

The propositions were as follows:

1. Clients who perceive themselves as having inner control over their daily activities will expect guidance and support from the nurse in response to their initiation of an interaction.

2. Clients who lack inner control over their daily activities will expect the nurse to act as an authoritarian figure who exerts control.

3. Clients who receive nursing care congruent with their expectations will feel satisfied with the nursing intervention, whether or not their problem has been solved.

4. Clients who receive nursing care that is perceived as divergent from their general expectations will be ambivalent about or dissatisfied with their care even when progress toward their goal has been achieved.

5. Clients who cannot identify their problems or who have no definite expectation of the care they will receive from the nurse will be ambivalent or dissatisfied with the care given.

DISCUSSION

The majority of clients in this study decided on their own initiative to seek health care at the Workship. For some clients, the effect of cumulative problems had created a level of stress with which they could no longer cope. Generally, clients saw themselves as independent and able to solve their own problems on a day-to-day basis, but when they contacted the Workship, they felt that they had lost control over the situation. This supports LeFeourt's contention that:

> If the locus of control is external, unrelated to one's own behaviors in certain situations and beyond personal control, he will perceive the situation to be more stressful.[6]

When these clients believed that they had obtained information that allowed them to resume control of the situation, their stress level was reduced, and they felt able to cope with the situation again. This suggests that it is important for the nurse to identify those areas perceived by the client to be strengths and to work with these. At the same time, the nurse must avoid behavior that indicates to the client that external control of the situation is being imposed by the nurse.

There was an atypical group of clients who requested external control of the situation by the nurse. These individuals exhibited lifestyle behaviors demonstrating a generalized lack of control over their own affairs. They did not perceive themselves as able to solve their own problems and sought an authoritarian approach from the nurse. When this was not given, they were less than satisfied with the client-nurse interaction. This suggests that at least at the initial encounter, nurses must be alert to the types of expectations that a client has of the health professional.

The way in which a client's expectations of the role and function of the nurse were met was of more importance in this study than was progress toward a stated goal. If a client recently discharged from a hospital expects the nurse to take his pulse and check his blood pressure, it may be important that she accepts these functions at the initial visit, even when the stated purpose is to support the client in an attempt to decrease an observed high anxiety level.

One critical function of the nurse was to listen to the client's feelings, fears, and ideas. The nurse was an informed listener, and it was this knowledge base that differentiated her role from that of a neighbor. Clients could view the nurse as a friend, but this did not detract from their image of her as a "professional." Friendliness was viewed as an asset because it made the nurse approachable, but her knowledge differentiated her from the usually accepted role of a friend. While the nurse was expected to be knowledgeable, she did not have an immediate answer to a problem. The important thing was that she was able to identify the resources that she would utilize before the next contact with the client. Thus, nurses were able to say, "I don't know the answer" without any loss of status, but they had to be cognizant of the many sources of information and alternative resources available to them in the community.

It is important for nurses to be alert for those clients who have had previous negative experiences with the health care system. While the number in this study was small, it would appear that one of their major concerns was that in previous encounters with health care personnel, they felt that they had lost control over the situation. They did not understand the doctor's orders or the explanation given related to their illness, so frequently the stress they experienced was severe. For these clients, the establishment of a trusting relationship was critical, particularly when the client was afraid that no one would give him information. This is where books and reference materials may be useful. The client can read the information for himself and then discuss areas not understood with the nurse.

Some clients who were referred by other agencies seemed to have difficulty in understanding the purpose of the nurse's visit. The nurse must be alert to the expectations of clients who have been referred by others. If the client has no clear expectations of the care the nurse will give, it is necessary to explore mutual goals and identify the nurse's role before nursing intervention commences.

This study demonstrated the need for the nurse and client to establish congruent goals. It also showed that for nursing care to be effective, the nurse must be sensitive to the client's expectations of her role and the activities in the nurse-client interaction.

REFERENCES

1. Leininger M: The phenomenon of caring: importance, research questions and theoretical considerations. *In* Leininger M (ed): Caring: An Essential Human Need: Proceedings of Three National Caring Conferences. Thorofare, NJ, Charles B. Slack Inc., 1981.
2. Glaser BG, Strauss AL: The Discovery of Grounded Theory: Strategies for Qualitative Research. Chicago, IL, Aldine Publishing Co., 1967.
3. Glaser BG: The constant comparative method of qualitative analysis. *In* McCall GG, Simmons JL (eds): Issues in Participant Observation. California, Addison-Wesley Publishing Company, 1969.
4. Mayeroff M: On Caring. New York, Harper and Row, 1971.
5. Ingram DR: Distance and the decision to visit an emergency department. Soc Sci Med 12(4):55–62, 1978.
6. LeFeourt H: Internal versus external control of reinforcement: a review. Psych Bull 65(4):206–222, 1966.

INDEX